WOUNDED TO
WARRIOR

HOW TO
PARTICIPATE
IN YOUR
OWN
RESCUE

TIFFANY OWEN

WOUNDED TO

WARRIOR

How to Participate in Your Own Rescue

Copyright © 2023 Tiffany Owen

All rights reserved.

Cover design by:

SpeakTruth Media Group LLC

Published by:

 SpeakTruth Media Group LLC

Special discounts for bulk purchases, sales promotions, fundraising, and educational needs, contact SpeakTruth Media Group LLC at order@speaktruthmedia.com.

ISBN: 979-8-9884573-2-9 *(pb)*

Printed in the USA

DEDICATION

To all of the people currently struggling in silence with PTSD, mental health issues, and addiction. And, to the families of the people who did not win their battle with addiction and/or suicide ideation. You are not alone. There is hope. God is still in the miracle-working business!

ACKNOWLEDGMENTS

I want to first thank God for putting such a strong desire in my heart at the age of six to write this book and for seeing me fit to walk through the fire and overcome. Nothing was going to stop me from being a vessel to further His kingdom in a mighty way.

I'd also like to acknowledge and thank my husband, Chris Owen, for loving me unconditionally, always seeing greatness in me, and supporting my dreams and goals no matter how crazy they sound.

Thank you to my children Collier, Jagar, Teegun, and Talon for loving me, respecting me at my worst, and being patient with me through my recovery.

Thank God for my mentors and friends Kristen Glass and Lenee Rogers for being a big part of helping to save my life.

Big shoutout to my #ATeam for cheering me on through this process and all my clients who have trusted me to partner with them on their transformation journey.

I also want to acknowledge my writing coach, Charlana Kelly. Without her lighting a fire under me, praying for me, and guiding me through the process of writing this book, it would not have happened in such a timely manner.

Lastly, I want to acknowledge all the people in my life who were a part of my trauma. I forgive you. I own my part, and I see you with compassion for what you, too, have gone through.

TO THE READER

Dear Friend,

It is no accident you are holding this book. I prayed for God to bring you into my life to help you be radically transformed into the person He created you to be. I want you to set your expectations before you start reading. Expect God to reveal to you the things that may need to be healed or acknowledged in your life.

Expect to have a different perspective about the people in your life who may be currently experiencing PTSD, mental health struggles, or the disease of addiction. Expect to be inspired and receive a new hope of what is possible when you apply what you learn from my book. Give yourself permission to think differently. Be open and curious with a growth mindset. Put your negative emotions, unhealthy habits, and mindsets that are not serving you on a shelf while you take this journey with me. You can pick them back up any time you feel like it.

If at any time you feel triggered as you are reading, take that as a sign that God is telling you something inside you needs attention and healing. If the triggers are overtaking you, please skip to the action step portion at the end of the book. This portion will give you tools that will help you process and heal as you continue reading my story.

God hears your prayers. My prayer is that by reading "Wounded to Warrior," you will learn how to participate in your own rescue and become the dominant force in your life.

Love,

Tiffany Owen

CONTENTS

FOREWORD

Romans 8:28 came to mind while I contemplated my thoughts as Tiffany's closest confidante. Tiffany and I have been together for thirteen years, filled with many ups and downs throughout. Every time we overcame a trial, we'd jokingly say, "That's another chapter for your book!" Tiffany knew she was supposed to write a book since she was six; however, we could never imagine it would be like the one you hold today.

I wanted to be part of this book in some way to share my thoughts and let you know that hope and change are possible. I'm writing as the person on the other side. The person whose loved one is struggling. The person who's spent an extended period praying with tears, wondering if God was punishing me, if God made a mistake, and if "it" was ever going to get better.

Well, "it" does and can get better, God doesn't make mistakes, and He's not punishing you. He's refining you in the process and qualifying you to help others who may be going through a similar situation.

At the time I am writing this, Tiffany has been sober for about seventeen months and is practicing DAILY everything she prescribed in this book. I am astounded at her level of commitment to her nonnegotiable daily routine. I have witnessed her become a totally different person by practicing what she preaches. I am in complete awe and have fallen in love with her all over again on a much deeper level. The things she writes down come to pass over and over again.

Tiffany is being radically transformed into the person God intended her to be right now. She is 100% committed to doing the work and she always takes personal responsibility for her part. So, if you're questioning and doubting at this moment, please stop. Give yourself permission to think differently. You don't have to know how or where your thinking will take you. Just do it. God will work out the rest.

One thing I know, God fulfills His promises and as I stated when I started, Romans 8:28 is the perfect promise to take hold of for your personal situation or loved one. "And we know God causes EVERYTHING to work together for the good of those who love God and are called according to his purpose for them."

Never doubt that God has your best interest in mind, and EVERYTHING works out for the good. Keep praying and believing. God has something amazing in store for you.

— Chris Owen, Tiffany's husband

Today, my mom is a vastly different person than she was during my childhood. As I am now in Australia, I have been watching her transformation from afar and could not be prouder of her. During my childhood and teenage years, my mom was quite unstable, due to the various forms of trauma she experienced throughout her life. I never knew what I was going to get from her, as she was constantly up and down using alcohol as a coping mechanism. I hold absolutely zero blame towards her, as she is simply a human being, just like the rest of us. She experienced horrendous events throughout her life. That being said, her trauma affected everyone around her, as she was not at peace with herself, nor was she able to regulate her emotions properly.

Moving forward, in the past year and a half, I have noticed a tremendous change in my mother. She is regularly happy and positive, and she is completely sober from alcohol, which benefits my stepdad, my little brothers, her friends, and, most importantly, herself. I could have never imagined that my mom would truly heal so drastically, but she has. I see a positive difference in her, more and more, every time I speak with her. She truly is an incredible woman. I wouldn't wish to be the daughter of any other.

— Collier Kosovich, Tiffany's adult daughter

INTRODUCTION

It has been said that the journey of a lifetime begins with *one step*. There are no hard and fast rules about when that step must occur (I'd say, the earlier, the better); it is just a requirement to begin. Once we commence our pathway, progress is often *two steps forward, one step back*, as many who have gone before us, mine included. So, the point can be made that the most important part of the journey and the steps you take along the way is to arrive at your destination of choice.

My advice to you is to choose life, healing, and victory. Be a warrior who overcomes the wounds, the abuse, and the self-loathing hatred that drives you to destructive behaviors that prevent your hopes and dreams from becoming reality.

From Wounded to Warrior is my testimony, my life, and my journey to a breakthrough that will hopefully inspire you to avoid the pitfalls of life's vicious cycles that hinder our progress to a life of love and joy.

My hope for you, as with every person I encounter, is freedom and a sense of power from within that releases you to be all God created you to be in the here and now.

While I share the pain of my childhood and the decisions of a broken heart that led to greater destruction, I also share the process of healing that broke the cycle. My pain has become my purpose of teaching, training, and coaching people like you as to how you can participate with God in your rescue.

Like me, I hope you will see your great worth and catch a vision for how you can help others break their painful cycle to realize their victory, too.

Be sure to connect with me on social media to share your own testimony about how my story helped you go from tragedy to triumph. Share the victories of how your dreams became a reality.

I'm cheering you on! I believe in you! I know you can live the life you desire with a little help from a friend.

So, let's be friends! Remember, as you read this book, you have a friend holding your hand and walking right beside you.

CHAPTER ONE

DEFINING MOMENT

Do you have a defining moment? One sets the stage for your deepest insecurities and fears. I remember *mine* like it was yesterday—now 33 years ago.

I heard the concept of a "defining moment" while watching the Dr. Phil Show about 20 years ago. A defining moment is a point in your life when you're urged to make a pivotal decision or when you experience something that fundamentally changes you. Not only do these moments define us, but they have a transformative effect on our perceptions and behaviors.

Everyone has defining moments that shape how they internalize, interpret, and react to events and situations for the rest of their lives. As Dr. Phil talked to his guests about their defining moment, I had a revelation and knew precisely when mine happened.

I was nine, living in Kentucky with my mom and her new husband. The incident instilled a fear of abandonment that was so strong I have held on to it into my forties. It was a fear that led to panic, insecurity, and self-destruction. Honestly, I am not even sure my mom knows how much this night affected me.

I went to bed like usual, with the TV on and the sleep timer set to go off after falling asleep. Yes, the TV had been putting me to bed for as long as I can remember. For some reason, I woke up and felt very alone. I walked into my mom and stepdad's room sometime after 11 p.m. to discover they weren't there. As panic started to set in, I quickly walked downstairs to check the rest of the house to see if I could find them.

Scared to death, my heart began to race as I frantically walked around the house searching for them. I was used to being home alone, but this was different. They didn't tell me they were going anywhere. I wasn't supposed to be alone. For goodness sake, it was the middle of the night, and I was only 9!

Heart racing, stomach hurting, and breathing panickily, I reluctantly checked the garage for their cars. If I opened that door and their car was gone, I would have to face the reality that I was alone in a new place where I knew no one. As I opened the door, I was devastated to confirm what I was already thinking. They were gone! They didn't tell me they were leaving. I had no idea where they were or when or if they would return.

I am pretty sure that moment was my first official panic attack. And it began defining every other moment in my life.

I ran to the sliding glass doors in our living room that went out to our back patio to watch the road for their car. Our house was two stories, and it overlooked a golf course. Between the golf course and my house was the road coming into the subdivision and a stretch of woods. I could see every car coming into the subdivision.

My stomach was hurting so bad. I didn't know anyone to call. I had moved with my mom from Texas to Kentucky after she announced that she was leaving my dad for another man. I didn't know my stepdad's family and was never given a phone number in case of an emergency. I felt like I had been abandoned. I stood at those sliding glass doors for what felt like an eternity. Every time I saw headlights, I hoped and prayed it was them coming home. Hope would spring up in my heart until I realized it wasn't them. As quick as hope came, despair flooded my heart again, over and over again.

My memory fades at this point. I can't remember the details of their return, but I know it was after many hours. It was probably around 2 a.m. when they walked through the door. I vaguely remember my mom acting like it was no big deal. My worry and anxiety were made out to be invalid. They acted like I was at fault because I got out of bed.

Sadly, there was no nurturing, love, or apology. What they did was say it wasn't a big deal. Maybe it wasn't a big deal to them, but to me, being left alone in the middle of the night set the stage for my debilitating fear of abandonment and rejection!

Have you ever felt abandoned or rejected? What are some insecurities that you struggle with? Have you ever thought about the root cause of those emotions? When did they start? What happened to you that caused you to feel that way? I bet you, like so many, have a defining moment from an early age that continues to shape you, your relationships, and your future.

I learned in my late twenties at a retreat I attended to save my third marriage, something that has stuck with me to this day. Yes! You read that right, I was in my late twenties and on my third toxic marriage. The retreat's theme was *"You Cannot Change or Heal What You Don't Acknowledge"* (author unknown). The retreat did not save my marriage or me as I had hoped, but that quote alone led me to dig deep into my heart as to why I was stuck in a cycle of victimhood and self-sabotage.

One of my intentions for writing this book and sharing my story vulnerably is to help you identify why you have fallen into a life shaped by a victim's mentality and self-destruction. At nine years old, I started feeling like a victim and stayed in that torturous mental prison for most of my life. I had many moments where God rescued me and gave me undeserving mercy and grace, but I kept returning to my old thoughts and behaviors. Why couldn't I stay rescued? What was wrong with me? Why was I reaping a life pattern of trauma, abuse, and "everything wrong always happens to me" reality?

The story I shared about being left at home alone was only one of my many defining moments. Reflecting on your life, one moment may stand out more than another. I have found that most of my traumatic defining moments are the ones I have suppressed the memories of into the deepest parts of my mind. Unfortunately, my experience over time has shown me these suppressed traumatic memories will continue to resurface if I don't identify and process them.

I have learned in the last few years that what you focus on grows! I am not sure I got that concept when I first heard it. At first, I thought it meant if you think about all the positive —

bam — you will have it in your life. Experiencing positive results in your life couldn't be easy, or everyone would be living a spectacular life. I was missing a big part of this concept. What you focus on grows. I wasn't just referring to the rainbows and butterflies I dreamed of having. It also meant that anything, even the negative, will increase if that is what I focus on daily.

My experience with trauma, horrible circumstances, and devastation goes way beyond being left alone at home. I will share more of that as you continue to read. For the sake of making my point to help you move past your negative defining moment, let's focus on my debilitating fear of abandonment and rejection. As a result of my experience, my belief became that "everyone who says they love me either leaves me or abuses me." I repeated this belief to myself continuously from childhood through my thirties. I went into every relationship with this expectation at the forefront of my mind. The thought pattern became my focus. And boy, it became a reality in my life.

I labeled myself "abandoned and abused" before entering any relationship. I let it sabotage any connection I had, whether it was family, friend, or romantic. I did not discriminate. If you encountered me, I forced you into that box no matter what. Honestly, no one had a chance. My walls were thick and high. I would be ready when it happened. I would not allow myself to get hurt, so I often sabotaged everyone before they had a chance.

I was clueless that I could have healthy connections if I changed my focus. My fear of abandonment got so severe I felt it in my body. I was so desperate for unconditional love, but I couldn't receive it when it was offered. I kept everyone at arm's length. I set them up to fail. And by doing so, I FAILED!

Here are some examples of how insecurity played out in my body. I must hold a pillow over my stomach when sitting, and I sleep holding a small pillow or stuffed animal. Another thing I do to make myself feel secure is putting my feet up off the floor and crossing my legs anywhere I sit. I am sure my husband thought this was so strange when we first got together, but he never judged or questioned me.

Holding and pressing something tight against my stomach makes me feel secure and safe. I guess it's the same as a child with PTSD or an autistic person sleeping with a weighted blanket. When my middle is exposed, I feel extreme discomfort and vulnerability. I think some of this stems from sexual trauma too. You can see how fear and insecurity defined me.

Maybe your defining moment has nothing to do with fear of abandonment and rejection like mine. Your defining moment may have something to do with sexual abuse, physical abuse, verbal abuse, falling into the trap of addiction, an eating disorder, terminating a pregnancy, being adopted, or giving a child up for adoption, being raised in a broken family, or growing up in poverty and neglect. I cannot name them all here, but you understand my point. I want you to know that I empathize with you and have experienced most of the circumstances I just listed. I feel your pain. I see you. I was you. There is hope.

I did not grow up attending church regularly, but I always knew something or someone bigger than me was protecting me along my journey. My parents took me to church occasionally, and I attended a couple of private Christian schools, but no emotional or spiritual experience was attached. Looking back, I recognize we were just spectators checking a box. Unfortunately, I did not grow up in a house with solid morals and values, and I was unaware of the relationship and spiritual connection a person could have with Jesus.

The good news is that God placed very special people in my life who would minister to me and plant seeds that would come to fruition at the right time. Has God put people in your life like that? Maybe you didn't notice them in the moment, but looking back, you know they were from God. He was showing me the whole time that I was not alone. I would never truly be abandoned or rejected if I leaned on my Lord and Savior. Oh, how I wish I could have genuinely felt that with my heart as I went through all the pain, struggle, and self-sabotage. If I had made that head-to-heart connection earlier in my life, I might not have turned to abusive relationships, drugs, and alcohol to fill the void in my heart.

I'm reminded of Hebrews 13:5! I may not have grown up knowing the Bible or learning about God's promises, but now I hang on to every promise like my life depends on it. I realize the importance of teaching my four kids about our relationship with Jesus when we accept Him as our Lord and Savior. After horribly failing at three marriages, I finally met my godly mate at 29. Chris has shown me what a true relationship with God looks like.

I have played tug-of-war with God most of my life. I would cry out to Him to save me, and He always did. However, I would quickly go back to old behaviors, patterns, people, and mindsets. He never failed to send me His rescue boat. I always climbed in only to jump right out a short time later. Chaos and abuse were like comfort zones to me and all I knew. Often, we become addicted to the familiar even when it has the potential to destroy our future, which is one of the biggest reasons people stay stuck. It seems easier to suffer in the known than step into the miraculous unknown that will dramatically improve our lives.

I have a tremendous desire to overcome my past. I also want to gain victory over my body being in constant survival mode. Through many years of counseling and trauma treatment, I have learned tools that empower me to overcome self-preservation mode. It's been a journey of convincing my body and assuring myself I am safe. Like me, you no longer have to live in survival mode; there is no threat. You can create, you can become—the unknown is safe.

Meditation has become an instrumental part of my healing process that has convinced my body I have a new mind and that I no longer need the protection I once did.

Your trauma is your trauma, whether it is big "T" or little "t" trauma. If you want to move forward and come out of the bondage of what happened, you must first start by acknowledging your defining moments. Is this hard and scary? Absolutely! It might be the most fearful thought to let go of your trauma and be healed. Fear is crippling. An acronym helped to change my perspective though. FEAR: Face Everything And Rise. We must shift our focus to what we desire and hope for in our lives, instead of what we don't want. Whether we are focusing on the negative or the positive, we will always possess exactly what we are looking at! And, here's the good news, we get to choose.

Here is something to think about. If we focus on all the things we do not want to happen to us, those things will begin to happen because that is where we focus. Have you ever been scared about having a flat tire? I used to check my tires every time I got into my car. If my low tire pressure light came on, I freaked out. The thought of getting a flat tire consumed me. Guess what? I experienced a lot of flat tires and low tire pressure warnings.

Instead of focusing on everything we do not want to happen, change the focus to all the amazing things we want and have in our lives. *Where you stare, you steer.* You will experience the great things in life that you are looking for when you practice fixing your gaze on your hope. It is not easy. It takes intentionality, but with consistency and time, your perspective will shift in miraculous ways.

It is time to do the scary thing and identify your defining moment so you can process it and begin healing as you move past and let go of what's holding you back from being the person God created you to be. Carl Jung said, "*Until you make the unconscious conscious, it will direct your life, and you will call it fate.*" In other words, until you consciously look at the unconscious trauma you are avoiding, it will trigger unwanted choices and behaviors.

What we visualize and internalize will materialize if we do it right. If you will first be open to change and give yourself permission to think differently, healing is possible. Remember, a decision is never a decision until actions are attached. If you make the decision to change, everything can change for you. The best part is you don't have to change what is outside. You change the inside, and the outside will follow.

I want to encourage you to stop waiting for your circumstances to change. If you are waiting for your circumstances to get better before you start making changes to anything in your life, you will probably be waiting for the rest of your life to get out of victim mode. You will continue to be in the mindset of "everything happens *to* me." I want to help you change your perspective to "Life happens *for* me!" I find so much comfort and security in the fact that I get to improve my circumstances, not the other way around!

Sheldon Kopp's words deeply touch my soul, resonating in a life-changing way, "Running away may relieve our anxieties momentarily, but lasting ease requires our turning toward what we dread most. In dealing with fear, the way out is *in*."

CHAPTER TWO

WHAT BOUNDARIES?

A boundary is simply a clear line that tells you/others where to stop, defining where one area ends and another begins. It's vital to establish boundaries. Without them, our lives are chaotic and ineffective at best. Do you lack boundaries? If so, have you ever thought about where your lack of boundaries came from? Do you have a problem saying "no"? Can you pinpoint a moment when not being able to say "no" set the stage for the rest of your life?

WHY I DID NOT HAVE BOUNDARIES

Today, I am very grateful I don't have an issue saying "no" and meaning it without explaining myself or feeling guilty. "A grown woman never has to explain herself," is something I live by now. Unfortunately, that was not the case up until I had a breakdown so detrimental, I tried to take my own life. I hope that will not be the case for you. From my rock-bottom response, you can see that boundaries are vital for your health and well-being. I'm thankful I learned the lesson, albeit the hard way.

Let me start by sharing where my lack of boundaries started. I believe it stemmed from being left alone all the time as a child. I craved attention and connection to fill the void left by my parents, not giving it to me. My cravings were so significant I would do anything to fit in and get attention. Alcohol became a huge crutch that helped me connect with people at a very young age. And I had zero boundaries when it came to alcohol consumption.

To begin with, my overwhelming need to be the center of attention was ignited early on in my life. I don't have many fond family togetherness-type memories. I was often left to my own devices starting at six years old. My parents were always gone either on trips or traveling for work. It became a family joke that I was changing my own diapers at 18 months old. I was "independent," so I guess my parents thought that was a win. As I reflect, I don't believe they did this intentionally or had any idea how it would affect me.

I was left fending for myself throughout the Summer and after school from first grade on. That innocent little girl had no idea what the lack of nurturing and attention would do to her as she got older. Yes, I was mature and smart for my age, but now, as a mother of four kids, I realize how much I had been neglected emotionally. I can't even imagine leaving my kids home alone at that age. Unfortunately, that was my normal. I remember feeling so mature and thinking I could do grown-up things.

Financial lack was not an issue, I had everything a kid could ever want. Possessions could never replace being told I love you or being hugged and kissed. My trauma was partly due to the lack of nurture, affection, and attention. The stage was being set for a lot of emotional instability that led to my addiction to alcohol and prescription drugs. To reiterate, I had no boundaries regarding anything that would change how I felt or make me feel seen.

MY FIRST DRINK

At 12 I discovered what alcohol could do for me. My parents had been divorced for a few years. My mom was working two jobs day and night to provide all the material goods she thought I wanted, and I guess she wanted to. I was always home alone at this point, and with no supervision, I began hanging out with older kids who were considered the "troubled crowd." I would end up with my best friend, who was a year older than me, at boys' houses where their parents weren't home either. I guess we were what was termed latchkey kids.

I first got drunk at one of the boys' houses. He had some 40-ounce beers hidden in his room. All five of us took turns taking drinks from the bottle. When it was my turn, I guzzled the beer instead of taking a normal sip, like I was dying of thirst. It went down so easily, and I remember thinking it was smooth. My craving for beer seemed unquenchable; I could not stop after the first drink.

It took a little while for me to feel the effects of the alcohol, but when I did, I remember it hit me hard. My vision was blurry, my speech slowed way down, and I couldn't get the words out that I wanted to say. Something inside of me wanted more of what felt like an out-of-body experience. Have you ever wanted more of a feeling that was dangerous, making you lose all faculties and coherence? Why would anyone want to feel completely checked out?

The crazy thing was when we made it back to my best friend's house, we had what felt like a very long conversation with her mom without her knowing we were intoxicated. How in the heck did she not notice? Realizing I had the ability to hide when I was inebriated opened the door for me to not fear getting in trouble for changing the way I felt whenever I got the chance.

I do not remember the ride back to my house. As usual, there was no one at home awaiting my arrival. All I can recall is laying down in the front yard and passing out for who knows how long. I was so relieved when I woke up, and my mom had still not made it home. I did it! I got drunk for the first time without getting caught! Did you get caught the first time you consumed alcohol or got high?

I DO NOT BLAME MY MOM

As I continue to share more of my story, I want you to know my experience of my mom is based solely on my perspective and reality as a child. I have learned that a person's perspective of reality does not always make it true. I want to be clear that I do not blame my mom anymore, and I have forgiven her for all the things I blamed her for that happened to me throughout my adolescence. I understand that she experienced major trauma of her own, which molded her into the person and parent she had to be to survive life. I have compassion for my mom instead of anger and resentment. I want to encourage you to forgive and let go if you are holding on to bitterness. By releasing the person who caused you pain, you free yourself, which is exactly what I did. Forgiveness was a major part of my healing journey, and it must be a part of yours too. There is no way around it!

A PRODUCT OF MY ENVIRONMENT

My lack of boundaries also stemmed from no one modeling them for me as a child. I never even heard of such a thing until I was in my late twenties while in treatment for a prescription drug addiction. I felt like my mom never paid attention to anything I did because I never seemed to get caught. In her defense, I showed no signs of being a troubled kid. I made straight A's, was self-motivated, and teachers loved me. I also kept the house clean (if I didn't, I would get yelled at, backhanded, or both), and I ensured I cared for all my needs.

My mom worked her butt off to support me. Even though she was never home, I now know she did her best to show me love. The more I was alone and not getting healthy attention from my parents, the more I desperately sought it in unsafe and unhealthy ways. I was determined to be noticed one way or another. I never said "no." I went right along with whatever the kids I was with were doing. I also found ways to drink or get high as much as possible. Changing how I felt would help me survive the pain of feeling like I wasn't loved and didn't matter to anyone unless I was "performing."

ADDICTION IS A DISEASE

I believe that I was born with the disease of alcoholism and addiction. With addictive behaviors, those "demons" awakened in me early in my life. It would be an ongoing battle I fought from that moment forward.

Has a lack of boundaries in your life caused you to do things to change the way you feel or put you in compromising situations where you didn't have a high self-esteem level to empower you to say "no" for fear of rejection? By the grace of God, I am sharing my story with you from a place of complete healing and deliverance. It has taken about 40 years, but I have finally become the woman, wife, and mother God created me to be. God's mercy and love have helped me overcome trauma and pain to inspire and give hope to those still suffering in silence. My pain is truly my purpose!

I love what Elizabeth Benton says in her book *Chasing Cupcakes,* "In order to be a part of the solution, I had to stop being part of the problem. I decided that I wanted solutions more than I wanted attention, and I had to start acting like it," (Pages 278-279).

NO FEAR OF CONSEQUENCES

Coming out of denial is the first step in recovery from the disease of addiction. Accepting this realization has been a lifelong process and a tug-of-war with myself. I took one step forward and three steps back, more times than I can count. Sadly, my addiction was not just to alcohol. I found myself loving the way prescription pills made me feel like a superhuman who could do everything necessary to have the energy to perform above and beyond for the love and attention I longed for.

For those of you who may be struggling or have had a prescription pill addiction, I want you to know there is hope and that you aren't alone! My addiction to RX medication started around age 17. A friend gave me one of her ADHD pills because I wanted some extra energy. I was a straight-A student on the drill team, Z Club, and Student Council, in an abusive, toxic relationship, and I worked most nights of the week at a local restaurant. I was very busy and trying to manage it all with perfection.

My lack of boundaries made it easy to say yes to anything without considering the consequences. I was hooked after the first pill I popped. The energy was amazing. Who needed boundaries? I could say "yes" to everything and get it done better than most people.

Addiction is progressive, I built tolerance very quickly. After only a few short weeks, one pill did not give me the same burst of energy. I would need more to get the same feeling. My friend handed them to me like candy for about a year until I took over 20 pills one night and accidentally overdosed, landing me in the ER with a toxic liver.

HISTORY OF PRESCRIPTION PILL ABUSE

I did not take pills for a long time after that. The overdose and time in the hospital scared me enough to lay off until my early 20s when I became a personal trainer.

I quickly realized I needed extra energy for all the things I said yes to and to perform at superwoman levels. I was a young wife with a husband in the military who was overseas on deployment. I had an 18-month-old daughter then, and I needed energy again. I also didn't want to feel fat and hungry all the time. My body had to be perfect! I was a personal trainer, after all.

I innocently discovered prescription diet pills when they became popular and available online. It seemed like everyone was taking them, with very little understanding of the risks or side effects. I honestly just wanted more energy and some help controlling my appetite. I built tolerance quickly again; one pill a day wasn't enough. Anxiety and depression were escalating. I didn't realize the pills contributed to those uncontrollable emotional outbursts. I couldn't function without taking a pill.

Fast forward to my mid-20s. I went to the doctor for severe back and hip pain. He gave me pain pills. I needed to perform. I needed to do as much as possible. I had no boundaries, and I couldn't speak the language of "NO." I was married for the third time to a toxic husband and had a 5-year-old daughter and a baby boy. I needed the physical pain in my back and hips to go away. I did not have time for pain or discomfort with everything on my plate. I needed the pills to make me feel better about myself.

I quickly realized *these* pills gave me an indescribable energy, a euphoria I wanted more of — I became hooked immediately! Why couldn't I be like most people who become tired when they take pain pills? I felt like super woman when I popped them every chance I got. It was a horrible double-edged sword. My self-worth came from how much I could accomplish. And taking those pain pills helped me get *a lot* done. I did whatever it took to get my hands on more pills. I "doctor shopped," looked through medicine cabinets whenever I went to someone's house. I justified my theft by telling myself, "It's okay, they would never miss a few pills." Most of the time, the bottles had been in the cabinets for months or years. My thought process was they weren't going to take them anyway.

At my lowest point, I was probably taking at least three to ten diet pills and/or pain pills daily! I'd break them in half to make me feel like I was making them last longer, but ended up popping one every 2 to 3 hours. I knew I had a problem, but I couldn't seem to get a hold of my out-of-control desire. Feelings of "no way out" flooded my heart and mind. As a result, my desire to kill myself to set myself free from this prison of addiction was through the roof. I was destroying myself, my marriage, and my children then. The marriage was never healthy, to begin with, but I wasn't making it any better. I continued the destructive cycle, reinforcing the false belief that whoever said "I love you" would abuse and abandon me.

My relationship with my husband became so rocky and tumultuous that he served me divorce papers, which I had no idea were coming. He was extremely passive-aggressive and non-confrontational. After I was served divorce papers, I quickly got my act together. I could do that very well if my back were against the wall.

I convinced him I would do whatever it took to get him back, and he gave me a second chance. The divorce papers were dropped, but I quickly reverted to old, unhealthy behavior. We ended up having three sets of divorce papers over a 2-year period. The back-and-forth cycle was torturous, more than I could handle emotionally and mentally. My pill problem and alcoholism ramped up worse than ever before. I wanted it all to be over.

How much more could I take? I was trying to figure out how to kill myself non-painfully. Maybe I could wreck my car to make sure I died, so no one else would be injured in the process.

My first suicide attempt at 16 didn't work. My overdose caused my kidneys to fail, but I didn't die. What else could I do to stop hurting myself and those I loved? Remember, I had no boundaries regarding what I would do to myself because I believed my body was worthless. I was worthless. All I did was bring pain to others.

My kids did not need a mom like that in their life. Thinking, "they would be better off without me," played on a continuous loop in my mind. I was more afraid of living than I was of dying. The madness had to stop one way or another. I had to do whatever it took to stop the pain and regain my family.

I did not want a third failed marriage, even if it wasn't healthy. My dad had been married five times, and my mom was on her fourth. I never wanted to be like them, but here I was, continuing the cycle. I begged God to save my marriage. I was so devastated by how my life was going that I felt like my heart was literally being ripped out. My husband told me that if I got help, I would get my family back. I needed to hear his words to figure out how to get help.

MY FIRST TIME IN TREATMENT

In 2010, I checked myself into a mental hospital and then a 90-day rehab facility. While at the mental hospital, I was blindsided by the third set of divorce papers. I was handed the papers by a stranger who snuck in through visitation. The walls were closing in on me, I fell to my knees and began crying uncontrollably. How was this happening? I was told that if I got help, I would get my family back, but the opposite was happening.

I am grateful now that I sought help, but at the time the devastation of being deceived by someone that I thought loved me seemed more than I could handle. God had a plan for me better than I could have ever imagined. Unfortunately, at that moment when everything was being ripped away as I tried to do the right thing, it did not feel like I would ever wake up from this nightmare.

About a year after I completed treatment, God blessed me with my godly mate. Even though I kept repeating a vicious cycle of abusive, toxic relationships, I secretly hoped God would bring the man He chose for me into my life. Surprisingly, I never gave up on finding true unconditional love. Each time a marriage fell apart, I cried out to God, asking Him to please bless me with the man He had for me. The prayer I repeated over and over was, "God, please bless me with my godly mate. Let me recognize him, and him recognize me without a doubt."

It was a miracle from God that I believed was possible. In spite of everything I had been through up to this point in my life, I had a belief and faith so strong inside of me that could have only come from Him and the people He put in my life along the way who planted seeds of hope in me, prayed for me, and spoke truth and life over me. I prayed with such a strong belief that I would thank God before that man came into my life like it had already happened. Mark 11:24 says, "*Whatever things you ask when you pray, believe that you receive them.*"

Chris and I married in December of 2010, and we got pregnant with twin boys in April. It was a little less than a year after I finished my 90 days in treatment and three months sober. Our story is amazing, and I look forward to sharing more of that with you later.

If you have been in the cycle of abusive relationships and constantly picking the same type of person repeatedly, I want you to know there is hope in finding the one that God has for you. Start praying that prayer I mentioned and, more importantly, start working on becoming the person God created you to be.

Finding my godly mate was only a stepping stone to breaking my destructive habits. I brought a lot of baggage and trauma into our marriage. I was not healed. I was still broken and had a lot of issues. The euphoric high I got from my new and magical relationship with the man who adored me and loved me unconditionally was short-lived.

GOD DELIVERED ME

My struggles with addiction were not over, and I continued to have many slip-ups. I never ceased praying for a miracle to be freed from my self-made prison of obsession and cravings. I always found myself wanting to take another pill to change the way I felt. Why wouldn't the cravings go away? Once, I took one pill the phenomenon of craving set in, and I lost all control.

It was a true miracle when I had a hysterectomy in 2011, solving my chronic pain issue. I had something called adenomyosis, which caused the pain in my back and hips. I was an addict, but it was huge. I had to be a willing participant in my own rescue. I had to put pride and ego aside and ask for help and support from my husband. I can now have surgery without the fear of getting addicted again. Chris and I decided long ago that he would keep and administer all the prescriptions I needed to take. Forever! And, I had to be honest with myself. I cannot take medication as prescribed; if left to myself, I will take more than I should.

If you are struggling with any kind of addiction, I want to implore you first to admit that you are powerless over whatever substance you are addicted to right now. Second, be honest with someone about your problem who you love and trust. Third, turn your will over to God and get help, which can look different for everyone. Be open and curious. Addiction is addiction; whether you are addicted to prescription pills, alcohol, narcotics, marijuana, pornography, food, or any other substance that is controlling you. There is a way out if you are willing to seek help.

I wish I could share right here that this was the end of my problems with substance abuse, but it was not. My lack of boundaries, PTSD, and mental health issues would wake my "addiction genes" back up when I let my guard down. I fooled myself into thinking I was different. I was cured. But for me, cross-addiction was very real. According to the Hazelden Betty Ford Foundation, the terminology refers to people with two or more addictions. I returned to alcohol. I had control for a little while until suddenly, I did not anymore. The disease of addiction is cunning, baffling, powerful, and progressive, and there is no cure.

Fortunately, I am sober now and in the best mental state I have ever been in my entire life. The past 42 years have been filled with trauma, tragedy, abuse, self-loathing, self-harm, and a roller coaster of emotional and mental health issues. The amazing news is that my life has also been full of miracles, answered prayer, and protection from God, even with a lifelong battle for my life to finally become the best version of myself that I would win! Are you at the bottom of a dark hole you cannot climb out of? Are you tired of being tired and fighting for your life? Are you a burden to your family and everyone you encounter? Hang on! There is a way out!

Let me share again from Elizabeth Benton's book *Chasing Cupcakes*. She wrote on page 153, "You have to be willing to let go of the problem and not cling to it simply because it's familiar or makes you feel justified in your lack of progress. You don't have to retreat into the familiar story of the problem." One of the first steps in getting my life together was to admit that I was a huge part of the problem. If you embrace this with a positive perspective, the good news is that if I am the problem, I need to change what is happening inside of me. I can control myself and how I respond to situations instead of reacting to everything with a defensive attitude and victim mentality. I have zero control over other people and most situations, but I completely control myself! There is true freedom in coming to that realization.

Did you know that the National Association of Mental Illness reports that 1 in 5 U.S. adults experience mental illness annually? There are so many people walking around who are battling their minds, and you can't always tell by looking at them. According to Mental Health America, the suicide statistics are catastrophic. According to reports, "Suicide is the

10th leading cause of death in the U.S. It is the second leading cause of death among people ages 15-24. More lives are lost to suicide than any other single cause except heart disease and cancer. In 2020, 12.2 million adults had serious thoughts of suicide, 3.2 million made a suicide plan, and 1.2 million attempted suicide in the last year. Those with substance abuse disorders are six times more likely to commit suicide than those without."

One of my many miracles and blessings was that I got to go to an amazing trauma-centered workshop at the facility, Onsite in June of 2022 after my final rock-bottom incident with alcohol and my fourth suicide attempt. It was absolutely life-changing on so many levels. I received healing and many tools I could use to help me manage the PTSD, depression, addiction, and anxiety I struggled with.

At Onsite, I learned that the external things we use to calm internal noise, discomfort, or stress are called *"medicators."* We all have ways we medicate, some healthy and some unhealthy. Unfortunately, it seems like many of the healthier ways people once dealt with stress were either taken away from us or no longer served the purpose they once did in taking the edge off our ever-increasing stress. Sadly, there has been an increase in and normalization of drug and alcohol use and abuse, in addition to process addictions like gambling and pornography. And let's not forget those sneakier addictions like food, relationships, shopping, scrolling, binge-watching TV, etc.

I'm so grateful today that God has delivered me from the phenomenon of craving alcohol and prescription pills, but that doesn't mean I don't still struggle with the lows of depression triggered by past trauma. There are still days I struggle. My defenses are often down when I am not feeling well or overly exhausted. The enemy tries to sneak in and start messing with my mind when I'm sick, tired, lonely, and/or angry. I started questioning my existence and my mission to help others. The old negative tapes in my head can start playing on a loop. I must pay attention and remind myself that feelings are indicators, not dictators. I must be vigilant to fight the enemy's lies in those moments.

Before I got sober, I would buffer my emotions with alcohol. Today, I don't have that option. I must feel the feelings, process them, and then, hopefully, sooner than later, use the tools I learned in treatment at Onsite to get out of the funk. It is very helpful to bring darkness to light immediately when these negative thoughts, feelings, and emotions begin to consume me. I have someone in place that I trust who I can reach out to and let them know what is going on. I do not need them to fix me or tell me it will be ok. I just need them to listen so I am not holding these feelings inside. When I verbalize what is happening inside me, the darkness loses its power over me.

If I'm feeling beaten down by outside circumstances I can't control, it can take a little longer for me to dig myself out of the hole I've crawled into. Often, when I'm in a state of trauma response, I freeze. My body goes into protection mode. I go into *shutdown* or *collapse mode.* I learned at Onsite that I'm immobilized and unable to move in this state. I can't say "yes" or "no" when I'm in this state.

In what's termed a "Dorsal state," consent is lost. Have you ever wondered why a person can't leave an abusive situation or when someone is being sexually abused once or multiple times, they cannot say "no"? There were many times when I experienced physical/verbal/sexual abuse I could not say "no" or leave the situation! I blamed myself and couldn't understand why I "let it happen." I was grateful to discover the reason. In this state of shutdown, the person is unable to consent. They can't say "yes" or "no"! Wow! Everything made more sense after learning this fact. Maybe, it wasn't all my fault.

We will never be completely free of circumstances, things, and people that cause pain, suffering, stress, anxiety, and hurt in our lives. Pain is part of life in our earthly bodies.

Life circumstances were part of what led to my final breakdown in 2022. The challenges left me hopeless enough to decide suicide was my best option. I'm sharing this because I want those struggling with the same issues as me to know I'm not completely cured; I still struggle. I just handle the struggle differently now than before.

The difference between now and then is I'm not medicating with alcohol, drugs, self-pity, avoidance, exercise, or food! I love my life, and my pain is my purpose. I am living to serve and help others as a health, fitness, and mindset coach and advocate for mental health. I have so many amazing clients and a community of fellow coaches who give me life and purpose as I help and serve others.

I am blessed with the tools I use daily and the non-negotiable boundaries I have set in place. I won't lie; it sucks feeling the feelings of a broken heart and other things out of my control. But I can't heal what I don't feel. So, today, I embrace the "suck" because I know it's temporary. Sometimes the temporary is long, and sometimes it's short. I don't think about suicide or alcohol as an option to cope anymore. Let me share some tools with you! The path to healing and wholeness isn't a straight line; it's a spiral. We often return to things we thought we understood, only to go deeper into the truth.

As you continue on this journey of trauma to healing with me, I pray you find hope, inspiration, and action steps to help you overcome whatever you may be facing.

CHAPTER THREE

I COULD NOT SAY NO!

SEXUAL ABUSE AND SEXUAL ACTIVITY AMONG CHILDREN AND TEENS

According to the Rape, Abuse & Incest National Network (www.rainn.org), "One in 9 girls and 1 in 53 boys under the age of 18 experience sexual abuse or assault at the hands of an adult. 82% of all victims under 18 are female. The effects of child sexual abuse can be long-lasting and affect the victim's mental health. Victims are more likely than non-victims to experience the following mental health challenges,

- About four times more likely to develop symptoms of drug abuse
- About four times more likely to experience PTSD as adults
- About 3 times more likely to experience a major depressive episode as adults

I am heartbroken but not shocked to share that according to the National Center for Health Statistics, "Over half of U.S. teens have had sexual intercourse by age 18."

At the age of 12, my first sexual encounter was with an 18-year-old. I did not think this was abnormal. It felt good to be wanted by someone. Does it still make it sexual abuse if I wanted the attention? Was it all my fault, or was it his fault, and was he taking advantage of me? These are questions I have battled in my mind since I realized that a 12-year-old and an 18-year-old having sex was not normal and not okay.

I did not have anyone telling me it was not ok. I have wrestled with the fact that I did not fight him off. I welcomed it. I had friends who were sexually active with their boyfriends. Granted, most of them were a lot older than me. My grandmother let me be alone with this young man. Surely, she knew what was happening or could happen. She did not warn me or tell me it was wrong. It had to be my fault. Was I sexually abused?

My heart breaks as I write those devasting statistics and recall my own experiences, but the information also helps me to understand why I have struggled with my mental health and addiction for most of my life. Knowing that there has been an underlying root cause to all the insanity and instability I have experienced was probably not all my fault, and I was not simply crazy, has helped tremendously in my healing and moving out of a victim mindset.

Do you ever feel like you are being defined by your worst moments? Do you struggle with extending grace towards yourself? Have you been in a situation where you were taken advantage of sexually by someone much older who should have known better, but you blame yourself because you did not say no or fight them off?

THE ROOT OF WHY I COULD NOT SAY NO

I was often left home alone, unsupervised by an adult, starting at the young age of 6. I don't have many fond memories of spending quality time with my parents or doing things as a family. They always seemed to be gone on trips or traveling for work. When they would travel out of town, I was left with a babysitter or my Nanny (my mom's mom) most of the time. This was my normal, but that normal would leave a void in my heart that longed to be filled by connection.

It was always joked about that I was changing my own diapers at 18 months old. I was labeled a very "independent" child, so my parents thought that was a win. Constantly being left alone during the day in the summer and after school, until my parents got home from work to fend for myself, starting in the first grade, made me feel like I was an adult. A first grader should not feel like they are an adult that can do adult things. I had no idea what this lack of nurturing and attention would do to me as I got older.

To give my parents the benefit of the doubt, I don't think they knew the repercussions. Yes, I was mature and smart for my age, but now, as a mother of 4 kids, I realize how much I had been neglected, especially emotionally. I can't even imagine leaving a child that young at home alone. On the other hand, I was always provided for financially and had all the things any kid could ever want. Things do not replace being told I love you or being hugged or kissed. This independent and smart little girl had no idea how something as simple as being unsupervised at such a young age would affect her ability to make good choices when it came to right and wrong and trusting others.

My trauma was beginning, and it would set the stage for a lot of emotional instability. I am extremely grateful that I acquired so much awareness at Onsite. I learned through my time in trauma treatment that I was in the early stages of codependency as a young child.

According to Onsite Journal, Volume Two, page 32, "Codependency is *a trauma related loss of self*, something that happens when our primary caregivers aren't emotionally available to give us the love and nurturing, we need. With the field of addiction becoming more understood in relation to trauma, it turns out that codependency is simply another coping mechanism that comes from growing up in trauma, just like alcoholism, drug abuse, or workaholism (or any other ism you can think of).

When caregivers don't show up in a way that could meet our emotional needs, children learn that the best way to get their needs met is to try and meet the needs of the parent (so the parent might have something left over for them.) Parents who can't meet their own emotional needs create children who attempt to be all things to all people.

These dramas are re-enacted repeatedly, the child trying to meet the needs of the parent (and to be hypervigilant in anticipating the needs of the parent) in the hopes that the parent will, in turn, meet the child's needs, see their hurting heart, and finally give unconditional love.

I longed for unconditional love way before I understood what it was.

In addition to trying to meet my parents' needs when they were present, I also tried to meet the needs of whoever I was with. In many cases, I would try to meet the needs and desires of older boys and sometimes men, which led to promiscuous behavior after my first sexual encounter. All it took was one time! In the moment of being manipulated into having sex at 12 with an 18-year-old, I felt loved.

Sadly, I mistook inappropriate sexual behavior for love. This would also play out in the many toxic relationships I would get involved in. I wanted to become all things for all people so they would show me unconditional love. If I had sex with them, maybe they would not leave me. Wow, that was a big burden to carry for me and the person I was trying to get to love me. It was clear I was raising myself and wasn't doing a great job.

WAS IT ALL MY FAULT?

I have been tormented by this question my entire life. I did not fight them off. I began drinking and using prescription drugs on a regular basis around the age of 12 after my first sexual encounter. I put myself in compromising situations where older boys and sometimes grown men could easily take advantage of me. It had to be my fault. How could that be sexual abuse especially since I did not say no?

There are so many times that I remember feeling powerless and I would freeze in the moment when I was being touched or coerced into having sex by these boys and men that clearly knew what they were doing. I was living in a constant state of fear and survival. When I am really scared, I do not think right. The attention and comfort I found in those moments where I was being touched, intercourse was being performed, and I was being told how beautiful and amazing I was, was a powerful force. It was a very dark and negative force that was all-consuming and controlling.

Have you ever found yourself in an unhealthy, dangerous, and compromising situation and you froze? You did nothing to stop it. You were paralyzed. You just let it happen and maybe even participated like you were having an out-of-body experience. Then afterward you beat yourself up and shamed yourself as you were the mastermind of the entire situation. Have you questioned if you were the victim or the perpetrator? If you have found yourself in a situation like mine or similar, stop blaming yourself, especially if you were a child and the person who did the unspeakable things to you was an adult.

It has taken me decades of torturing and blaming myself to finally come to the realization that I was the victim. I was a child who did not know any better, with a very distorted view about love and healthy relationships and connections. If an 18-year-old took advantage of my daughter sexually when she was 12, there is no way I would blame her. Why did it take me so long to stop blaming myself? I was absolutely disgusted and ashamed of myself because I honestly cannot even tell you how many times, I did not say no to having sex with whoever made me feel even the slightest bit special and loved in the moment.

Now, as a parent, I know with my intellectual mind that I was a victim of sexual abuse on countless occasions as a child all the way up to the age of 18, but I do not always feel that in my heart. Have you ever said to yourself, "If they really knew everything I had done, would they still say it wasn't my fault? Would they still think I am a victim?". Maybe the counselors did not hear me when I said I was blacked out and drunk or that I just lay there and did not say stop. Was I still a victim if, at the moment, I was feeling loved and wanted and I enjoyed what was happening to me?

Of course, it was not my fault! I was a child. They were often over 18 and always much older than I was. I understand this in my head, but I often do not feel it in my heart. I am missing the head and heart coherence. If I label myself the victim, do I lose the power that I thought I had in those moments where I would find myself in a worst-case scenario? If I admit that I was a victim of these men who just wanted to use me for sex and pleasure, then that would mean I never meant anything to anyone. I was just a sexual object that could be used and then thrown away, which was the case in every one of these tragic encounters.

Yes, that must be why I go back and forth between being a victim and not being a victim. I must continue to educate myself about why I respond and react the way I do. Knowledge is power and will help me heal.

HEALING CAN BEGIN WITH KNOWLEDGE

We have three parts of our nervous system that influence how we will respond to something. We can make better decisions when all three parts of our brains work together. Unfortunately, when we are experiencing trauma, stress, and triggers, we cannot get all three parts of our nervous system to wire and fire together. The three parts include the ventral stream, the sympathetic nervous system, and the dorsal stream.

The ventral stream processes visual information for the purpose of visual perception. This is where the connection between people and our environment takes place. We were born for connection. Coregulation, possibility, and social safety are established in the ventral stream.

The second part of the nervous system is called the sympathetic nervous system. According to the Cleveland Clinic, "Your sympathetic nervous system is a network of nerves that helps activate its "fight-or-flight" response. This system's activity increases when you're stressed, in danger, or physically active. Its effects include increasing your heart rate and breathing ability, improving your eyesight, and slowing down processes like digestion." In this state, we only see danger. We are in motion first, then we think later. People tend to be very impulsive in this state and say things they do not mean when feeling threatened. It is your body's way of trying to protect you, but it can be a very volatile state where we say things like, "I want a divorce. I hate you. Leave me alone. I never want to see or talk to you again. Etc.". I spent much of my life constantly in this state of self-preservation, and a lot of self-sabotage happened.

The third part of our nervous system is the dorsal nervous system. According to the Very Well Mind, "The vagus nerve's dorsal side responds to danger cues. It pulls us away from connection, out of awareness, and into a state of self-protection. In moments when we might experience a cue of extreme danger, we can shut down and feel frozen, an indication that our vagal nerve has taken over." I had to be in this state during all my trauma with sex and abuse. The Dorsal state is a state of rest and digestion. We experience a shutdown emotionally and sometimes even physically. Fainting or collapse can occur in these instances. All consent is lost. We are unable to say no, immobilized, and unable to move.

Learning about this was my aha moment. I was mostly in a dorsal state when I lay there and could not say no when I was being taken advantage of sexually as a child. I had confused my inability to say no with consenting and participating with what was horrifically being done to me. I was in complete dorsal shutdown. It was not my fault. It was my body's way of protecting me, even though that was not what it felt like at the moment.

Tragically, I would continue thinking that letting anyone who wanted to have sex with me was normal, and it felt like the love and attention that I so desperately desired because I was not getting it at home. This would eventually lead to me having feelings of disconnect and numbness in most of my relationships as a wife, mother, and friend. When God brought true unconditional love from my husband into my life, I could not receive it and feel it with my heart.

I had no doubt my husband and my kids loved me. I saw it when I would catch my husband gazing at me for no reason at all. The unhealed part of me would get a little irritated and defensive. My protectors would show up in full force, and I would start asking him why he was staring at me. What was I doing wrong? Did he think I looked fat? Was he about to accuse me of something? The negative stories in my head would automatically start running rampant. It was exhausting not only for me but also for him. How long would he continue to gaze at me with this look of awe in his eyes before I pushed him away to the point he may not fight for me any longer?

Knowing and feeling are two very different things. At that point in my life, I had so much healing left to do, and I would have to endure several more valleys, bottoms, and self-destruction before I could have true head and heart coherence. It would take time, work, and much more battling with the old me before the numbness and walls around my heart could start coming down. Thank God that Chris never gave up. He never stopped reaching out for hugs, kissing me when I would shrink back, or telling me how beautiful I was and how much he loved me. His consistency and perseverance would eventually pay off, and God would bless him with the godly wife he deserves.

Brene Brown's quote is so applicable to my life and may also be to yours, "We cannot selectively numb emotions...when we numb our pain, we also numb our capacity for joy, gratitude, and happiness." My hope for you is that you can identify the root causes of your pain and self-destruction. It is only then that the healing process can begin. When you do the work to heal, you begin to experience the joy, gratitude, happiness and love you so desperately have longed to feel. You won't be numb anymore, and you won't need those walls around your heart anymore.

Brene Brown also said, "You will grow and find intimacy when you share your pain as well as your joy with others." I am convicted to share my pain with you as well as my joy, so I, too, can grow, continue to heal, and find true intimacy in every area of my life.

Consider this play on the word intimacy: "Into Me See." As we share our life's story and the pain we overcame as we healed, we find the healing we have always longed for over the years.

CHAPTER FOUR

ABUSIVE ATTENTION WAS BETTER THAN NO ATTENTION

FACTS ABOUT TEEN DATING AND VIOLENCE

I believe change must begin first with awareness. We live in such a self-proclaimed "I am too busy" society we can easily miss what may be happening in our homes, especially with our children. So many parents are consumed by their busy work schedules, kid's activities, their own mental health and/or addiction issues, marital problems, and just simply getting by that they miss the warning signs of their teenager being in an abusive and toxic relationship. I fell into these scenarios as a teenager living with a very busy parent trying to make it and get by the best she could.

These facts about teen dating violence from *DoSomething.org* should concern everyone and reveal areas of our lives and others we need to be aware of in case we come in contact with someone who needs help.

1. Roughly 1.5 million high school boys and girls in the U.S. admit to being intentionally hit or physically harmed in the last year by someone they are romantically involved with.

2. Teens who suffer dating abuse are subject to long-term consequences like alcoholism, eating disorders, promiscuity, thoughts of suicide, and violent behavior. (I have experienced all of these).

3. 1 in 3 young people will be in an abusive or unhealthy relationship.

4. 33% of adolescents in America are victims of sexual, physical, verbal, or emotional dating abuse.

5. Females between the ages of 16 and 24 are roughly three times more likely than the rest of the population to be abused by an intimate partner.

6. Violent behavior often begins between 6th and 12th grade. 72% of 13 and 14-year-olds are "dating."

7. 50% of young people who experience rape or physical or sexual abuse will attempt to commit suicide. (The first time I tried to kill myself, I was 16 and in an abusive relationship).

8. Only 1/3 of the teens who were involved in an abusive relationship confided in someone about the violence.

9. Teens who have been abused hesitate to seek help because they do not want to expose themselves or are unaware of the laws surrounding domestic violence.

HOW MY FIRST ABUSIVE RELATIONSHIP BEGAN

By the time I was 15 years old, I had been looking for love and attention in all the wrong places since the first time I was taken advantage of sexually at age 12. I seemed to be attracting boys who were experiencing their own forms of abuse and trauma in their lives. Often, victims attract abusers, and abusers have typically been victims, so the cycle plays over time and time again. I saw my abusers as who I thought they could become and who I wanted them to be. I did not see them for who they really were.

I was naturally attracted to older boys. My dad was 22 years older than my mom, so that seemed normal for me. I met many of these boys at parties where much drinking and pot smoking happened. Most of the time, the night ended in drunken, blackout sex. Of course, I wanted a boyfriend, but they just wanted sex for the night. They were quickly finished with me after I gave them what they wanted. Until one night, it didn't end in sex for one night. He latched on to me, too.

He became dangerously jealous and controlling very quickly. In an odd way, this felt good to me. This negative attention was attention, nonetheless. It filled a void in me. I became addicted to him, and he became addicted to me. I believed this had to be love. He loved me so much that he had to know what I was doing and who I was with every minute of the day. Wow! He cared about me.

I had had other short-term relationships. It was very short term because once they got what they wanted, and I got super clingy, things ended very quickly. This time was different. I will call him Max to protect his identity. I am certain he has his side of our story, and his reality is true to him. My goal is not to blame him. I want *you* to know how dangerous it can be when two broken people try to be in a relationship. I was 15, and Max had just turned 18.

I had known who he was since I was in middle school. I had always thought he was so cool and good-looking. I never thought that he would give me the time of day. I was very wrong. All it took was a party with a lot of alcohol and pot and being alone together long enough for him to talk me into having sex with him in the back of his truck. I said no many times until I finally gave in to him. In the back of my mind, I knew that was all he wanted, and once I gave it to him, he'd be done with me.

To my surprise, his jealousy and control over me were so strong that we stayed together until I was 23 years old. The entire eight years were a tumultuous disaster of breaking up and getting back together, him cheating on me, and so much verbal and physical abuse.

THE WARNING SIGN AND RED FLAGS

If you are reading this, and can relate to anything that I have shared, I hope this is your wake-up call. I want you to know that you deserve more, and you are worthy of someone who loves you unconditionally, as it says in Ephesians 5:25, "For husbands, this means love your wives, just as Christ loved the church. He gave up his life for her." It is possible. I have that kind of husband now. If you are waiting for a sign, this is your sign.

Recognizing the warning signs of an abusive relationship is the first step to opening the door of your seemingly inescapable self-made prison. Whether it is you in the abusive relationship or someone close to you that you think may be in an abusive relationship, there are key warning signs that will help you identify if it is time to get out or help someone who may not be able to see the signs for herself because she is so beaten down with zero self-worth that she stays because she thinks she deserves it.

One of the first things that happened in my relationship with Max was extreme controlling behavior. He would constantly question me about who I was with, what I was doing, what I was wearing, how long I would be there, was anyone "checking me out", and so much more. I would have to ask permission to do anything; if I didn't, I would experience extreme consequences. He made me feel like I did not have the ability to make good decisions. Max would camouflage his controlling behavior by over-emphasizing his concern for my safety.

Another huge red flag was Max's overwhelming jealousy and possessiveness. If I was not at school or work, I had to be with him or wait for him at his house. This was the time of pagers. We did not have cell phones. If he paged me and I did not respond immediately, Max would blow up my pager, and then when I would finally get to a phone where I could check in with him, I was instantly accused of doing something I was not supposed to be doing.

Do you feel like it's always your fault? Do you ever just take the blame for everything because that's just easier than trying to defend yourself? Abusers do not take responsibility for their problems, blaming others (usually the victim) for almost everything. It seemed like I was constantly being told, "You made me mad, you made me do this, or if you had not done this, I would not have done that." Most of the time, I would apologize incessantly, hoping he would stop freaking out on me. I did this so often when I did nothing wrong that I became a chronic apologizer to everyone.

I constantly defended myself and apologized for things I did not even do. I cannot count how many times I was accused of cheating on him. I never cheated on him. Even if I wanted to, I feared what he might do to me or the other person. On so many occasions, we would be driving down the road and would stop at a red light, and if I turned my head in the direction of someone who happened to be a guy, I was instantly accused of checking him out. He would say, "You are checking that guy out. I bet you want to f… him." I could not even look at another guy without being accused of this. I was terrified of looking in the wrong direction or at the wrong person.

Isolation from my friends started happening very early on in our relationship. I was involved in the school drill team and other social clubs and had an awesome friend group. My girlfriends came from great families that often loved me like I was their own because they knew I was not getting that kind of nurturing at home. I was in high school and supposed to be experiencing high school things. I should have been going to sleepovers, parties, and school functions, spending time with other girls my age, but I wasn't. I missed out on so much.

I was always afraid to do anything I was invited to do because I was scared Max would accuse me of cheating on him or worse, he'd threaten to leave me, and then I would have to experience my heart being ripped out from the trigger of the pain and fear of abandonment. Constantly putting my friends off and not showing up to everything they invited me to eventually led to them not inviting me anymore. I would slowly lose my connection with some amazing friends. Your abuser may be alienating you from your friends and your family. They try to keep you away from your loved ones because your loved ones may tell you to leave him because he is not good for you.

Max would bad-mouth everyone that I hung out with. He told me that they hit on him or tried to have sex with him. I would later find out that he was the one hitting on my friends and trying to sleep with them. The first time I found out that he had sex with one of my very best friends in the woods while we were all at a party together absolutely crushed me, and it set the stage for not being able to trust anyone who said they were my friend.

The verbal abuse was the worst. It has taken me decades to have any self-worth and not see myself as all the horrific names he would call me. I was constantly called a slut, bitch, whore, crazy, psycho, stupid, fat, and countless other degrading things. I think the verbal abuse left me way more scared than any of the physical abuse I endured.

Are you in a relationship with someone who has extreme outbursts of anger, and it seems to come out of nowhere? Is there sometimes physical aggression involved when this happens? If this is happening to you, it is likely you are in an abusive relationship. It is not always physical touch or action towards you.

I always walked on eggshells because I was terrified of making Max mad. These highly charged, aggressive outbursts could be dangerous, scary, and escalate quickly. His aggressive behaviors included using looks, gestures, or words to intimidate me. All he had to do was look at me with this evil, judgmental, and accusing expression on his face, and I knew I was in trouble. I would have to defend myself and be very careful to say the right things so he would not fly off the handle.

His angry outbursts also included throwing or smashing things, punching walls, or destroying property. So many times, I tried to call someone for help, and he would grab the phone out of my hand and throw it. Once, he threw my car keys at me so hard they stabbed me in my leg and left a scar. Some other examples of his physical violence were smashing things on my head, spitting in my face, grabbing and squeezing my arms so hard it left bruises most of the time, head butting me, or throwing me across the room or down to the ground.

Your abuser may not be physically harming you. Is he harming himself to manipulate you into feeling sorry for him and to prove to you how much he loves you? One of the scariest instances of this in our toxic relationship happened a couple of years into our relationship. I have flashbacks of this horrific moment often.

We were in the middle of one of our many breakups. He was a very heavy drinker. That night, I think he may have been using more than alcohol. He came to my house late that night after a screaming fight that started on the phone. He always accused me of messing around with other guys. I would not let him in the house because I feared what he might do to me, but I could not stop him. He broke down my back door and quickly made his way inside.

I was screaming. He was yelling. It got bad fast. I cried hysterically, yelling, "You don't love me!". This flipped a switch in him. He forcefully shoved me down the hall, entered my kitchen, and grabbed the largest butcher knife he could find. As I lay on the floor sobbing uncontrollably, he took the huge knife and sliced his arm multiple times. Blood started pouring out, going everywhere. I panicked. He snapped out of his anger and got a towel to stop the bleeding.

I was an emotional wreck; I could not drive him to the hospital. He ended up driving himself, and I rode with him. He immediately began concocting a story for us to tell his parents and the doctors so no one would know that he really did this to himself. It was amazing how fast he could get it together to create a lie to cover his tracks. Of course, I had to reassure him that I would go along with everything he said because he would surely make me pay if I didn't. He was a master at coming up with lies. In fact, most of what he said was a lie.

Have you ever felt like you were crazy and are losing your mind? If you are in an abusive relationship, gaslighting by your partner can take those feelings to the next level. According to Dr. Tatkin, who wrote an article for *Reader's Digest, The Healthy*, "Gaslighting is a major form of emotional abuse and is a term that's used to describe when one partner brainwashes the other to question their own sanity or the reality of the world around them. "It's a particularly heinous tactic to misdirect, lie, and deny any truth to another person by making them doubt their perceptions, memory, and sanity," says Dr. Tatkin. "If your partner uses gaslighting to escape from being found out, that should be a deal breaker."

There were countless warning signs and red flags from the very start of our relationship, but I was only 15 years old when we got together. I had no idea what a healthy relationship looked like. I could go on and on with examples of what you should watch for if you are questioning whether you are in an abusive relationship. It is easy to turn a blind eye to the warning signs God may give you or a loved one may tell you they see from the outside looking in.

Try not to get angry or defensive with the person in your life that you know cares about you and is coming to you with fear and worry about what they see happening to you in your relationship. They may or may not be right, but if you know they are truly coming to you from a place of love and genuine concern, listen to what they say. Be open to seeing your situation through the eyes of that person. It is so much easier to live in a place of denial, but what if what they are telling you is true? What if them sharing their concerns with you could save your life?

I will leave you with one more characteristic of Max, that was a constant problem that led to so many bad fights. He was extremely hypersensitive. He was always easily insulted, taking everything as a personal attack and blowing things out of proportion. This did not just happen between us. He was like this with everyone, especially his parents. He was always in "fight" mode and ready to take anyone on that he felt was questioning or judging him. He would use very intense intimidation to get someone to back down and go along with whatever he said to justify his behavior. Wanting always to fight everyone is not a healthy way to live.

STOP BELIEVING THE LIE THAT IT'S NOT THAT BAD!

Do you say, "It's really not that bad!" or "I deserved it!"? Are you constantly questioning yourself and your sanity? Is it hard to stay upset with the person who is abusing you because they always come to you with tears and emphatic apologies and promises that they will never do it again? Is it easier to believe that they are sorry and will never do it again than having your fear of being alone become a reality?

This was me for most of my life.

Getting out of denial, naming our trauma, and accepting our current reality is some of the hardest work we will ever do.

It is scary to admit that you are in an abusive situation. If we admit it to ourselves or someone else, then that means we must do something about it.

In *Onsite Journal, Vol. 3*, Scott Peck says, "It makes sense why we tell ourselves it wasn't that bad. Because if we were to admit that it was bad, we would need to shift our perspective, maybe get mad at someone, or set a boundary. We might have to come to terms with what happened."

I know how terrifying and hard it can be to leave an abusive relationship. The sad truth is they probably won't change. It will probably happen again, and each time the abuse happens, it will get increasingly worse, making it more difficult to leave because you have zero self-worth left. Please tell someone safe what is going on. Be open to what they have to say, and let them help you before it's too late.

CHAPTER FIVE

WHY WOULDN'T THEY STOP BEING MEAN TO ME?

SUICIDE STATISTICS

According to the *American Foundation for Suicide Prevention*, "Suicide is the 12th leading cause of death in the US. In 2020, 45,979 Americans died by suicide, and in 2020, there were an estimated 1.20 million suicide attempts." Sadly, I am unsurprised. I became a statistic for the first time at 16 years old.

I believe it is important to educate yourself on the issues that lead people to commit suicide and the warning signs. Learning what to watch for in yourself or someone close to you could save their life or your own.

According to *Mayo Clinic*, suicide warning signs or suicidal thoughts include:

- Talking about suicide, making statements like "I'm going to kill myself," "I wish I were dead," or "I wish I hadn't been born."
- Getting the means to take your own life, such as buying a gun or stockpiling pills.
- Withdrawing from social contact and wanting to be left alone.
- Having mood swings, such as being emotionally high one day and deeply discouraged the next.
- Being preoccupied with death, dying, or violence
- Feeling trapped or hopeless about a situation
- Increasing use of alcohol or drugs
- Changing normal routines, including eating or sleeping patterns
- Doing risky or self-destructive things, such as using drugs or driving recklessly
- Giving away belongings or getting affairs in order when there's no other logical explanation for doing this.
- Saying goodbye to people as if they won't be seen again.

- Developing personality changes or being severely anxious or agitated, particularly when experiencing some of the warning signs listed above.

Warning signs aren't always obvious and may vary from person to person. Some people make their intentions clear, while others keep suicidal thoughts and feelings secret.

Suicide is on the rise in our culture. We all need to pay attention to our family and friends with tendencies toward these signs. I can identify with most of them and remember the despair I felt. Many are suffering in silence. Maybe you can identify warning signs in yourself or another person. Suicide ideation was something I struggled with starting at the age of 15. It is sneaky and can feel like it is coming out of nowhere. No matter what, don't remain silent. Either get help for yourself or reach out to the one whose behavior you recognize these signs in.

WHY I FEEL COMPELLED TO SHARE MY EXPERIENCE WITH SUICIDE IDEATION AND ATTEMPTS

Have you ever thought to yourself? I could never do something like that to my loved ones. How could they do that?

They are so selfish. What were they thinking? Or how did I not know they were feeling this way?

First, if you've thought of suicide or attempted suicide, I want you to understand that you need to talk with someone about your thoughts and actions. Like me, you need help working through whatever issues and experiences drive you to want to end your life.

If someone you loved committed suicide, it is also not your fault. You may have noticed some irregularities or been unable to reach them, but the fact that they chose to do what they did is not your fault. Remove that burden from yourself now. Please! It isn't anyone's "fault."

In my experience, I was overtaken by emotional and mental torment that stemmed from more than one thing. One minute, I was fine; the next, I wasn't. Then there were other moments: my struggles with my mental health, my current traumatic/abusive circumstances, PTSD, battle with addiction, or pure exhaustion from trying to live life on life's terms overtook me. I was just too tired to keep fighting.

My purpose in sharing my personal experience with four suicide attempts over the span of the age of 16 to 41 is, first, to give hope and inspiration to those who struggle. More importantly, I want them to know they are not alone, and they are not bad people. Life doesn't have to be a constant battle where you are a prisoner of your own mind and circumstances.

I also want to offer introspection to those who don't understand why someone would try to hurt themselves or take their own life. Especially when it seems like so many people love them, and they have so much to live for. I want to offer you a different perspective so you can have compassion for those who do not have any fight left in them.

I never once thought I would be hurting someone who loved me when I tried to take my own life because, in my unstable mind and momentary insanity, I was a burden to everyone who loved me. At that moment, the only thing that went through my mind was how much they would be better off without me. The thought that they would all be better off without me played in a continuous loop in my head.

In sharing my most torturous mental moments, I hope I can offer you a different perspective into the mind of someone who is unable to fight the mental battle and torment that overtakes a person when they make that decision that they just can't go on any longer. It is absolutely devasting for all parties involved. It is tragic, but there is hope and healing. There is a way out.

God saved me all four times that I tried to take my own life. I was not sure why at that moment, but now I know why.

He would not let me die. He had a plan for me, and if you are thinking of ending it all, God has a plan for you, too. Trust me! Suicide is not the answer. Healing is possible. Coming out on the other side of this mental hell is possible.

How do I know? I know because I made it to the other side. I now feel with my whole heart that I am responsible for sharing my experience, strength, and hope with those struggling in silence. If that is you, you are not alone. You are not crazy. You are not broken and irreparable.

My pain is my purpose. Your pain can be your purpose, too. I love and live by what Ed Mylett says, "God doesn't call the qualified. He qualifies the called!" By sharing my struggles with hopelessness, darkness comes to light and the stronghold loses its power over me. So selfishly, I must share or risk going back to those thoughts that took me down multiple times. "Though no one can go back and make a brand-new start, anyone can start and make a brand-new ending," said Carl Bard.

SOMETIMES I HAVE TO LOOK AT MY PART

Have you ever found yourself trapped in self-pity with emotions running high and everywhere? Have you ever felt like no matter what you did, it would never be good enough, especially for the people you wanted some love and attention from the most? Have you ever asked yourself, why won't they stop being mean to me? Why do they hate me so much?

These were the questions that would play over and over in my head. I didn't understand why my mom and Max were always so angry with me. Nothing I did ever seemed to be good enough. I just wanted them to love me. No matter how hard I tried to make them happy, it never seemed enough.

Before I get too far into my story, I want to clarify that I no longer blame these people for my irrational emotions and impulsive actions. As I have done the work in my healing process, I have learned that I have a part in everything in my life. I realize that may be hard to accept for some people, especially depending on where they are in life. I got angry when I heard my psychiatrist at my first treatment center tell me this.

We rarely see our part when we are amid our trauma and pain. We can only see that we are a victim. Every victim needs a villain, and every victim also needs a hero. It can be easy to find that villain when it seems like everyone in your life is out to hurt you. It isn't always easy to find the hero. We often overlook the fact that we can be the hero of our own story and save ourselves from the torture and pain we are going through.

I am by no means saying this is an easy process. It is just something I would like you to think about.

Trust me, I have spent most of my life blaming everyone for everything that happened to me. How could I possibly be to blame when I was clearly the victim? It is rarely easy to take responsibility for our part in what happened to us. In accepting our part, we would have to look in the mirror, which leads to us having to work on ourselves. That can be more painful than the pain we are going through caused by others.

There was so much healing that happened when I started coming out of denial and coming to terms with the fact that I did play a part in the times that I was a victim. Hear me out! I get my power back by taking responsibility for my part in every life situation. I can evaluate myself and hopefully learn what not to do if there is a next time.

By owning my part in my mom and Max being mean to me, which led to my first suicide attempt at 16, I somehow got a sense of control and compassion for them, which helped me forgive them. Forgiveness is powerful and freeing. Forgiveness releases me from the hate that binds me to the person that hurt me. They stop taking up space in my head. They no longer consume me or control me or my reactions. I can move on.

That does not mean I must continue a relationship with them, but forgiveness allows me to release them into God's hands.

I strive to be more like Christ daily in every area of my life. To live a Christ-like life, I must forgive like He has forgiven me repeatedly. He forgives me when I don't deserve it. He forgives me when I ask for forgiveness, and even commit the same sin right after I ask Him to forgive me. Colossians 3:13 says, "Bear with each other and forgive one another if any has a grievance against someone. Forgive as the Lord forgave you."

MY FIRST SUICIDE ATTEMPT

I was 16 years old and an emotional wreck most of the time. I was excelling in school. I always made straight A's, making it hard to see how much I struggled mentally and emotionally. Most of the time, when a kid is going through something traumatic or using drugs or alcohol to self-medicate, they are not making good grades.

I had been in an abusive relationship with Max for at least a year. The emotional abuse had gotten so bad that I felt like I was dying inside, and my heart was constantly being ripped out of my chest most days. I cried all the time. I freaked out all the time. Most of my days consisted of chaos and drama. Peace and security were not emotions that I had ever experienced.

My mom was married to her third husband, and my dad was married to his fifth wife, who was only 12 years older than me. I did not seem to have a solid place in either of my parent's life. I was in the background, caring for myself and doing my own thing without adult supervision.

I was in my sophomore year of high school and had a job at Applebee's as a hostess. I was not only working most nights of the week and on weekends, but I was on the drill team at school. I was in all honors classes, on student council, and involved in Z Club (a community service organization). I strived to make straight A's because my self-worth was wrapped up in how much I could accomplish and how perfect I could be so I could get everyone's approval and praise.

On the outside looking in, someone could easily assume I was managing very well, considering my parents were never around and always preoccupied. I was always home alone or at Max's house. In my parents' defense, they probably weren't worried about me for the same reasons no one else seemed to be worried. I was not getting into any trouble, and I was working while making impeccable grades.

I clung to Max like a leach, probably sucking his life out because I was so needy for attention and affection. He had his own struggles and issues. He was not equipped to handle mine. We were two emotionally volatile teenagers who knew how to push each other's buttons, and we took everything out on each other because of the hurt that was going on in our home life. I would fly off the handle with emotional outbursts, and he would fly off the handle with extreme anger and violence. We were a recipe for disaster.

I do not really remember all the details leading up to the moment I decided I could not take anymore. I seem to be good at forgetting traumatic experiences and shoving them down so far that I have trouble remembering them. Shoving these details down and not being able to recall them has delayed my healing process.

It all happened so fast. There wasn't any planning or premeditation. I can't remember wanting to die leading up to this moment. My body and mind seemed to be in constant fight mode, just trying to survive the emotional rollercoaster I seemed to be on daily. It was exhausting, always on guard, waiting for the next time I would be accused of something or called horrible names like whore, bitch, slut, crazy by Max, or spoiled brat by my mom.

I felt like they hated me. Why were they always mad at me? Why could I not do anything right? Why did Max's love and attention only last for short moments of time? Why didn't my mom want to be around me? Why didn't she say I love you or hug me? Why did I always seem to make her so angry? What was wrong with me? Why couldn't I do anything right? Why did everyone who said they loved me leave me and/or abuse me?

I had to be the problem. I was the common dominator. The only thing that would help everyone was if I wasn't alive anymore. In my mind, at that moment, that was the only solution I could come up with to stop the pain of them being so mad at me. I was not good for anyone, and all I did was disappoint and make everyone mad, who I loved.

I was at home, and my mom was home for once. We got into an argument. I can't remember what it was about, but if I had to guess, it probably had something to do with my fighting with Max. It was very common for him to accuse me of something. I would lose it and start defending myself in a panic, begging him not to leave me. My emotions would escalate quickly, and the uncontrollable crying and yelling would start. It was the kind of crying where you hyperventilate and fall to the floor, holding my head in my hands, feeling like I was dying.

Something inside of me shifted quickly. Max hung up on me. My mom was ignoring me at this point. Who would blame her? I was so irrational and distraught that there was no chance of having a productive conversation. I was done. I could not take the pain anymore.

I walked into my bathroom, saying to myself repeatedly, why won't they stop being mean to me? I repeated that, and "everyone would be better off without me" on a loop until I convinced myself I was doing them a favor. I was saving the people I loved so much from the pain of being associated with me. I needed to take my life because I wanted to save them from me.

I could not see past this moment of temporary insanity. The problem was that this moment of insanity did not seem so temporary to me. This was my reality. I had to make it stop. I found a bottle of Aleve in the bathroom. I wasn't sure what it would do to me, and I didn't care. Self-harm seemed to be my only escape. If the pills didn't make me die, maybe they would at least make me sick enough for them to feel sorry for me and start showing me love and attention again. This was my only option.

I did not hesitate long. It all happened so fast. The bottle of pills was full. I poured as many as I could swallow at one time into my hand. I quickly put them in my mouth, drank water, and swallowed them all. I was all in at this point. There was no turning back now. I might as well keep going until all the pills were gone to ensure something awful would happen to me. I poured the pills into my hand and swallowed until the entire bottle was gone. There had to be at least 100 pills in the bottle.

I did not know what would happen next. I wasn't really scared, either. A sense of relief came over me because now my attention was on what I had done to myself, not them hating me anymore. I would take any relief I could get.

I went to bed with my eyes swollen shut from crying for so long. I prayed that God would let me go to sleep and not wake up. I was too tired to go on. I had no fight left in me. I just couldn't handle anyone being upset with me anymore.

To my surprise, when I woke up the next morning, nothing had happened to me after taking that enormous number of pills. I had to live another day. I had to force myself out of bed and put one foot in front of the other. I felt heavy and dreadful. Why didn't anything happen? How could I survive this mental torture another day?

God had a bigger purpose for me and a lot more life for me to live, but I didn't see that or want it the morning after I took all those pills. Was my mom going to treat me like she hated me and thought I was a horrible, spoiled brat? Was Max going to leave me? Did he still think I was some crazy slut? These questions and insecurities consumed me.

I did end up having severe consequences from my suicide attempt, but they didn't happen for a few days later. Around the third day after my breakdown, I started having excruciating back pain and overpowering nausea. I felt like my head was going to explode. I called my mom to tell her, but I felt like she thought I was being overly dramatic and making it all up. She told me to go to the doctor if I felt that bad. I always took myself to these kinds of appointments because she was busy or working.

Shortly after making it to my appointment, the doctor discovered I had gone into acute renal failure. I was immediately admitted to the hospital. No one knew that I had tried to take my own life a few days before. I told no one. I came up with the story that I had been taking a lot of NSAIDs for menstrual pain. This seemed to work because no one ever knew I had done this to myself.

My hospital stay lasted about a week before I turned a corner, and my body miraculously started healing without drastic measures being taken. The most traumatic part of my stay at the hospital was my mom not being there very much, and she never stayed one night with me while I was there. What was wrong with me? Why didn't she love me? I would continue to ask myself those questions until I was in my 30s.

Luckily, I was blessed to have my best friend's mom stay a few nights with me. I am sure she felt sorry for me, and I am very grateful that God placed many people like her in my life along the way that stood in the gap for the lack of parental love and attention I experienced growing up.

The doctors never found out what really happened, and I never told anyone. I'd be fine. Everything would be fine. I could handle this on my own. No one needed to know. I didn't want anyone to get angrier and more disgusted with me than they were, so I held onto that secret for a long time.

My body would heal, but my mind would continue to fall further and further into self-pity and victimhood. My situation with Max would only get worse. My use of alcohol and drugs would increase. My negative relationship with my mom continued to have a stronghold on me. How was I ever going to stop hurting? When would the emotional pain and torment go away?

Unfortunately, this would not be the last time I tried to take my own life. It is devasting to write that I attempted suicide three more times over the course of the next twenty-plus years. I have lived most of my life more afraid of living than dying. Death seemed like such a relief from the hell I was living on this earth.

HOW MY MINDSET BEGAN TO SHIFT OUT
OF WANTING TO DIE…

I have realized that once you stop fighting for what you want and need, what you don't want will take over. Whenever I felt like I did not have any fight, God would whisper to me, "Keep going. You can do hard things. Fight just a little longer, just for today. I will carry you when you feel like you can't keep going. You will survive, and it will be for My purpose."

I heard Damon West say something when he was being interviewed by Ed Mylett that made me feel Holy Spirit chills all over my body. He said, "You don't have to win every fight, but you do have to fight every fight." Something inside me shifted at that moment. I had to show up. Winning wasn't the defining moment in the fight. Showing up for the fight and giving it all I had was where the strength, courage, and determination would grow.

Everything changed when I:

1. Stopped blaming everyone else for my problems, pain, and suffering.
2. Took responsibility for my life and choices.
3. Decided life happened *for* me and not *to* me.
4. Decided to be the dominant force in my life.

5. Decided to do whatever it took to be the woman God created me to be, no matter how uncomfortable I must get in the process.

6. Decided to get in the lifeboat that God kept bringing me instead of watching it pass by me.

7. Stopped making excuses, and I started following through with the commitments that I made to myself.

8. Started declaring daily that everything always works out for me.

I believe if you can take these steps, everything can change for you, too.

CHAPTER SIX

I NEVER WANTED AN ABORTION

I'M NOT FINE

I am fine. It's fine. Everything is fine. How often have you told yourself and others that lie, hoping it would be fine if you just kept saying it? Does "I'm fine" ever actually mean "I'm fine"? In most cases, if we are honest with ourselves, it absolutely does not mean we are fine.

Saying "I'm fine" can be a way to cope with and buffer what is really going on. It is another form of just trying to survive and get by amid our pain and struggles. If we say "I'm fine" enough, then maybe it will be true, and what we are avoiding will just disappear.

Have you ever felt this way? Have you said it so often that you eventually convinced yourself that you can move forward without addressing the issue that you aren't fine about? I have been doing this most of my life about all the traumatic things in my life that I didn't think I needed to process and heal.

Despite what many of us grew up believing, sucking it up and brushing it off isn't always the solution. Sweeping things under the rug is a recipe for disaster. Stuffing your feelings and emotions may subside the hurt and emotional torment for a little while, but eventually, that volcano will erupt. It normally happens at the most inopportune time in your life.

I have learned that there are no good or bad emotions. There are just emotions. We don't have to label them one way or another. Every one of our emotions provides us with information. Our feelings can tell us a story about our lives and can help inform and navigate us through a healing process that will better equip us to move through our overwhelming days.

My default has been I am fine for a very long time until I realized it is okay to respond to someone asking you, "How are you?" with something other than "I am fine or good." Why do we tell people we are if we don't feel good? Why do we feel we can't tell them what is happening?

Next time someone asks you how you are, especially if it is someone you love and trust, tell them if you aren't okay. You may be surprised that most people have no idea what to say; if you don't tell them, you are fine. It is like we go around asking people how they are all day long, but we never take a moment to really stop and hear someone's true feelings.

I have had someone completely disregard my response when I told them I really wasn't doing great. They continued to talk like they never heard what I said. Are we listening to hear, or are we listening to respond? Really think about that before you ask someone how they are doing. You may be the only person who hears them, and you could impact their lives by showing you care.

I say all this to begin sharing my traumatic experience with abortion for the first time. I have pretty much shared openly and publicly everything I have gone through without any shame or fear of what others think. I'm always vulnerable, sharing with radical boldness to help, inspire, encourage, and give those suffering in silence hope. I want people who are struggling to know they are not alone.

The topic of abortion is the only thing I have hesitated to share because it is so controversial, and I have been telling myself it was no big deal. It really didn't affect me. I was fine, but now I realize maybe I have not been fine.

HOW I GOT PREGNANT AT 17

I was 17 years old and still having an on-again, off-again toxic relationship with Max. We would break up and stay apart for a month or two, then run into each other and immediately get back together. Things would be pretty good between us for at least a couple of weeks, and after that, the violent fighting and Max's narcissistic behavior would be like it always was.

We were addicted to each other in the most unstable and unhealthy way. We brought out the worst in each other but couldn't stand the thought of being without each other. We were the textbook definition of an abusive and toxic relationship.

We were never careful when we had sex. In true transparency, I didn't care if I got pregnant. We wanted to get pregnant because then we would have to be together forever. Sadly, I thought if I got pregnant, he would never leave me or abuse me again. He would have to stay with me, and we would live happily ever after.

Things seemed to be going great between us this time. We talked about wanting a baby together all the time. We would never tell anyone, but we were trying to get pregnant. That seemed to be the answer to all our problems.

Our relationship quickly turned violent again, and we ended up breaking up like we always did. He was off sleeping with other girls, and I turned to a lot of drinking and using pills to get high worse than I ever had before. I was putting myself in very compromising situations. I didn't care about anything, especially myself.

This is very hard for me to write because I am ashamed that I did not care enough about myself or my body to say no. I would have sex with whoever tried to have sex with me in most cases, especially if I was under the influence. I used sex (even unwanted sex) and attention to fill the void of abandonment and not being loved unconditionally by anyone in my life.

A few weeks after Max and I broke up, I went to a party and got extremely intoxicated. Before the night was over, I ended up sleeping with a boy who I thought really liked me, and I liked him too. After that night, it quickly became very clear that he only wanted me for one thing, which wasn't a committed relationship.

He ignored my calls, and I took a hint and moved on. I moved on to missing Max and wanting to get back together with him. It was like I was addicted to his control and jealousy he had over me. Attention was attention, and I did not care whether it was negative or positive. I craved it.

We had only been broken up a couple of weeks before we decided to get back together and try again. I found out I was pregnant shortly after that. We were trying, after all, so I immediately took a pregnancy test when my period was late.

We were both elated when the test was positive. We fantasized about getting married, having the baby, and what we would do to make it as a young couple. Max told his parents, and they were surprisingly supportive. We were going to do this! We could, for sure, make it work and be happy with their support.

I was afraid to tell my mom, and I really didn't have to right away because I wasn't even living with her anymore. She was in a relationship with a man who lived 45 minutes away, and she was always going to stay with him, so I was home alone all the time during my senior year of high school. My mom's best friend invited me to live in her guest house, so I wasn't always staying home alone. It was easy to hide from my mom.

Max, his mom, and I went to my first doctor's appointment, where they did an ultrasound. We were so excited to see the baby. We seemed to be blissfully happy until the ultrasound showed how far along I was.

Max and his mom quickly started doing the math with the dates on the ultrasound that established how far along I was, and they came up with, I must have gotten pregnant when we broke up. I didn't have a chance. They had made up their minds that the baby couldn't be his. Without hesitation, he broke up with me immediately and called me degrading names. Now, what was I going to do? Once again, my whole world came crashing down around me.

I went from being pregnant at 17 with love and support from my boyfriend and his family to being the biggest whore they have ever met in a matter of minutes. It didn't matter that he was sleeping with God knows how many girls while we were together and while we were broken up. There was a double standard, and I had no defense.

The doctor clarified that I was so early into my pregnancy that the due date was only an estimate at best. Max and his mom only heard what they wanted to hear. Max was free from taking any responsibility, and I was the villain in this story. I always seemed the villain. Everything was my fault. Once again, I wasn't good enough.

I HAD NO CHOICE

Have you ever felt like your life was just flashing before you, and you were completely numb the entire time, simply going through the motions and barely surviving? Have you experienced that feeling where you can't speak up, and even if you had the words or the energy to say them, they wouldn't come out no matter how hard you tried? Have you felt like you were having an out-of-body experience where your reality felt like one big, long nightmare that would never end?

After we found out the baby was possibly not Max's, my whole world felt like it was over, but I couldn't bring myself to try and end it all because all that did the last time was make me sick, and the pain of living was worse. Suicide wasn't the answer this time. How was I going to move forward? What options did I possibly have?

My mom still didn't know. I hardly ever saw her anymore because she stayed with her boyfriend, who lived out of town, and I was living with her best friend. I was scared to tell her. How could I possibly tell her? I didn't even feel comfortable telling her that I started my period when I was 12 years old. Telling her I was pregnant and wasn't positive who the father was felt like the most terrifying thing ever.

I have blacked out most of this traumatic time, so I will do my best to recall it the way it happened. My memory may not be completely accurate. I will share what my memory will allow me to share from my perspective. The other parties involved, including my mom, could have a completely different version. My goal is not to make her or anyone else a bad person. My goal is to share my experience as I remember it to enlighten those who have not gone through this and to help those struggling in silence to not feel alone.

From the time of my first doctor's appointment to when my mom showed up at my door to tell me what we were going to do about my predicament, it was mostly a blur. I couldn't tell you how many days had gone by. It seemed like it all happened fast, though.

There was no arguing. I didn't have the life left in me to fight my mom on this. I had zero support. I had no plans. The guy I slept with at the party avoided me and showed no interest in having a relationship with me, much less a baby. I had to do what she said. I had no choice.

I had been accepted to the University of North Texas. I was supposed to go off to college soon and become something. I wasn't sure what that something was. I had no drive left in me. My life felt like it was over. I was lost with no hope and felt completely abandoned and hated by everyone.

My mom said she would handle it. There was no discussion involved in this decision. I just did what she said.

She made the appointment, and we traveled to Louisiana, where the nearest abortion clinic was. We lived in Texas.

I was ashamed and petrified by the thought of having to tell all the people I had shared that I was pregnant with and that I was no longer pregnant after I had the procedure. What would they say? What would they think of me? I had told many of my friends at school, and I also quit the drill team because I had every intention of having the baby. They were going to wonder why I wasn't pregnant anymore!

My first appointment at the clinic seemed surreal. The drive was an hour long to get there, and a complete and uncomfortable silence filled the car. I just wanted this nightmare to be over now. Shame, guilt, and remorse consumed me, but I also was relieved.

The clinic was a normal-looking brick building with a full parking lot. The staff was extremely friendly, and the waiting room was filled with women of all ages. This appointment was not the actual procedure. They did some bloodwork, counseled me (I have no idea what they said), and set up a time for me to return in a few days to terminate the pregnancy.

The nurse who did my bloodwork was the daughter of my mom's friend. We were surprised to see someone my mom knew at the clinic. She was loving and non-judgmental. I was grateful for her attempt to have compassion and care for my well-being. The experience was tolerable and quick. I hated that we had to drive all the way home and return. That was more time I had to suffer the mental torture of anticipating what would happen.

I guess the waiting period was intentional to give the person time to really think about what they were about to do so they could change their mind. I knew changing my mind just wasn't an option for me. It had to be done. There was no turning back. This was just one more thing my mom had to get me out of so I didn't ruin my life.

THE DAY OF THE PROCEDURE

I can't recall what time or day of the week it was. I only remember bits and pieces. I have blacked out most of this day, and maybe that is why I have been telling myself that it was no big deal. I am fine. I just did what had to be done. I have been telling myself for decades it did not affect me.

We walked into the clinic. It was packed. I assume there were designated days the clinic performed abortions, and everyone there that day was there to terminate their pregnancy. We were all in the same boat. No one made eye contact with anyone else. Most of us were staring off into space or looking down at the floor with numb expressions on our faces.

They called my name, and I walked back to the room guided by a nurse. I was handed a gown and told to get undressed and sit on the table. The first thing that they would do was an ultrasound to confirm how far along I was. This is a moment that burned into my mind. This was one of the only moments of this day I remember vividly. This was when I found out the baby was Max's, but it was too late.

As I looked at the monitor while the ultrasound was being done, I got sick to my stomach, and my heart skipped a beat. I saw the baby. I saw the heartbeat. I saw that the baby was measuring eight weeks and five days. I was further along than the first doctor had told me. There was no way it wasn't Max's baby.

I had no fight left in me. I didn't say a word. I just looked at the monitor with a numb and disconnected feeling. I felt like I was in an alternate reality. This didn't feel real. The doctor came in and explained what would happen next, and I just nodded my head, and then it began.

I laid back, opened my legs, and stared at the ceiling as the doctor inserted the device inside of me. The sound is something I will never forget. It sounded like a vacuum, literally sucking the life out of me. There was some cramping and discomfort, but that was nothing compared to the horrible suction sound that took over the room.

Before I knew it, the life inside of me was gone. The procedure was shockingly fast. It pains me to think of how easily a precious miracle created by God can be terminated with such ease and quickness. This was the end of a life I so desperately wanted. Gone in an instant. What were my consequences going to be? How was I going to live with myself and what I had done?

A nurse told me to get dressed, and I was escorted to a recovery room where I would have to stay for a few hours for observation before I could go home. I was taken to a room packed full of women on cots who had just gone through an abortion. No one talked. No one looked at anyone else. We all lay there in discomfort with mental and physical pain until they told us it was okay to go home.

We were all going home to different scenarios where we would most likely suffer alone and silently with what just happened. I wondered if these women had support. Were they going back to an abusive relationship? Had they brought themselves there swearing they'd never tell a soul about what they just did? Were they relieved? Were they sad? Did they have other children? Were they worried God was going to punish them and they would never be able to have children after what they had just done?

HOW I WAS ABLE TO MOVE FORWARD

Do you ever completely move forward and heal from terminating a life that God created? Could I forgive myself? Could God forgive me? If you have gone through this, maybe these are questions you have asked yourself.

If you can relate to my story, maybe you are still living with daily regret and beating yourself up for choosing not to have the baby. I cannot speak for others who have had to make this painful decision, but I can tell you how I have moved forward and gone on to have four beautiful children.

I will not lie to you and say what I did consumed me with guilt. That may have been because I stuffed the day that I went to the clinic down so far, almost like it never happened. I did not process or deal with it until I was well into my 30s. I was completely numb to the fact that I had had an abortion for many years.

I had convinced myself it was the right thing to do. I had no choice. It all happened so fast. At that moment, I had no fight left in me to argue with my mom or even think about raising a baby by myself, unsure of who the father was.

Even though it has taken me a long time to feel it, I have always believed God loves me unconditionally. If I repent for my sins and ask for His forgiveness, it will be given to me. Ephesians 1:7 says, "In him we have redemption through his blood, the forgiveness of sins, in accordance with the riches of God's grace."

I hang on to my faith and find reassurance in knowing that God will continue to love me no matter what. Despite what I did, God still blessed me with four children. I do not feel like He punished me or that I deserved to be punished. I also forgave myself.

I could not change what I had done at 17 years old, but what I could do is move forward by accepting and receiving God's grace and forgiveness for having an abortion. I could also use this painful time in my life as my purpose and a way to further God's kingdom by sharing my story to give others hope.

We all have two choices when we go through something as tragic as something like having an abortion. We can punish ourselves by living in a mental prison of replaying what we did repeatedly in our head, or we can forgive ourselves and turn our pain into our purpose. I choose daily to turn my pain into my purpose; there is so much freedom in doing that and living a life to serve.

CHAPTER SEVEN

The Cycle of Abusive Marriages and Divorce Begins

I BECAME A STATISTIC

There are many unfortunate statistics about the effects on children who come from divorced homes. I never wanted to be a statistic. I was determined never to get a divorce and be like my parents. Somehow, I believed in true love, and that marriage meant forever and could last forever despite what I witnessed with my parents.

Have you ever said to yourself, "I will never be like my parents!"? I was certain I would not repeat their pattern of divorce and multiple marriages. My mind was made up. I would do whatever it took never to get a divorce. That was not enough to keep me from doing exactly what they did.

In an article entitled, *13 Saddening Children of Divorce Statistics for 2022* by Marija Lazic on www.legaljobs.io, "37.6% of all marriages in the US end in divorce. 85% of people get divorced because of a lack of commitment. Children with divorced parents are twice as likely to attempt suicide. Teenagers whose parents divorce are more likely to experience mental health issues."

Unfortunately, I also fell into a statistic I found published by *Psychology Today*, which revealed, "Research shows that children of divorce are more likely to experience a divorce themselves. The statistics vary, but one study by researchers Paul Amato and Danelle Deboer indicated that if a woman's parents divorced, her odds of divorce increased 69%, while if both a husband and wife's parents divorced, the risk of divorce increased by 189%."

I want to give you a little history of my parents so you can better understand my family dynamic. My dad was 22 years older than my mom. If I recall accurately, they got together when she was about 16 years old. She had left home before finishing high school. My mom worked at a restaurant where she met my dad, who was almost 40 years old. That just seems crazy to me.

My dad had already been married and divorced twice with four children, two from each marriage. I do not know all the details, but they eventually got married and were married for several years, at least before my mom had me.

My parents traveled a lot with work. I do not have many memories of being with them because I was always left with a babysitter or my grandmother (my mom's mom). From what I can remember, they stayed married for about 16 years.

I have vivid memories of them arguing all the time. They ended up divorcing when I turned eight years old. My mom left my dad for another man, who she quickly married after their divorce was final. She was now on marriage number two.

My dad would go on to marry two more times. He was married five times in total. His last wife was only 12 years older than me. It was tough for me to have a stepmom who was so close to my age and over 30 years younger than my dad.

I was being raised to believe divorce and remarriage were normal. My mom would go on to marry four more times. If you were on the outside looking in, I was destined for divorce. I did not have a chance.

MY FIRST MARRIAGE OF THE FOUR

Have you ever been ashamed of something but also grateful for it at the same time? Have you ever stayed in a situation that you should have left a long time ago because you were fighting so hard not to repeat the patterns of your parents because you wanted to leave a different legacy for your children, only to end up doing exactly what they did? How could you shift your perspective and use what you were once ashamed of to greatly impact and help someone who may be exactly where you used to be?

That is exactly what I have done. I have shifted my perspective on the topic of divorce. Not all situations are created equally. Not everyone needs to stay in a marriage at all costs. Sometimes, people need to get out of a bad marriage because God has their godly mate waiting for them after they get through the storm when they do the hard thing they said they would never do.

I ended up marrying Max even though he was abusive. We got back together about six months after I had the abortion. We never talked about it, but he made me pay for it throughout our four-year marriage. I was 18, and he was almost 21 when we got married.

We had a horrible argument that quickly turned physical the night we got married. Nothing had changed. All the promises of how much he loved me and would never hurt me again were gone when we said, "I do." It didn't matter, though, because I would never leave him. I would never get a divorce like my parents. Maybe I could love him enough to change him into the husband I thought he could be.

I have discovered the very hard way that no matter how hard I try, I cannot love someone into being the person God created them to be. They are who they are. I want to encourage you to pay close attention to any red flags you see early in a relationship. Those warning signs are that person telling you exactly who they are. Unfortunately, most of the time, after you marry the person, their character defects will only get worse.

Max had joined the military, so we were not together during our first year of marriage because he was on his first deployment. I will not go into too much detail about our marriage because that could be a book. Just know the verbal and physical abuse got worse with each passing year.

I got pregnant with our beautiful daughter while we were stationed on the Marine Corps base in Hawaii, and I gave birth to her there at one of the military hospitals right about a month after 9/11. I prayed that God would bless me with a baby girl, and He answered my prayer shortly after we started trying to get pregnant. Maybe if we had a baby, things would be different.

Max was scheduled to go on deployment shortly after my daughter was born. After his deployment, he could get out of the Marines, so I went ahead and did an early dependent return to return home to Texas so I would not be by myself with a new baby. I lived with his parents for the last year and a half of his time in the military.

You would think he would stop being jealous and accusing me if I was at home with a new baby living with his parents, but the fights were just as bad over our long-distance relationship. They were worse because he was extremely insecure about not being there to monitor my every move. If I didn't answer the phone when he called or if he heard an unfamiliar voice in the background, he would freak out on me. I was constantly on edge and defending myself.

I thoroughly enjoyed my time with his parents. They were like the family I never had but always wanted. I loved hanging out with them. Even though I was exhausted by always worrying about Max being mad at me, I found security in living with married parents who seemed to love me and my daughter.

I have blacked out a lot of this time from my memory. There was so much crying, yelling, and worrying that I experienced daily because of my toxic and abusive marriage. He was the textbook definition of a narcissist. Despite how he treated me, I was determined to do whatever it took never to get a divorce. It would all be okay if I could just do better and stop making him mad.

As I said earlier, I could write an entire book on just our marriage, so I will fast forward to how it tragically ended. God rescued me! I begged God to save my marriage with everything inside of me. I knew God hated divorce, so I hoped He would save my marriage. God answered my prayers, but not by keeping me in this dangerous relationship. I truly believe that had we stayed married, I would have died. I would kill myself, or Max would do something to me or maybe even himself.

One Friday night, Max picked a fight with me, and everything quickly turned into being all my fault. I didn't even know what I had done this time. He stopped answering my calls and didn't come home for three days. I was scared to death that he was in a ditch, dead somewhere. I called a friend hysterically, crying, and she finally told me that he had been cheating on me and coming to her house to drink alcohol with her husband instead of going to AA meetings to get help for his binge drinking problem.

I went to the gym Monday morning, where I worked as a personal trainer, and he called me after I had just reported him missing to the police. He acted like I was crazy for being upset and told me he had just been hanging out with a friend fishing. I couldn't argue with him or prove he was lying. I could never prove that he was lying. He was an excellent liar who could always flip things into being my fault.

I knew that I had to get help and get out of this marriage. I didn't want my daughter to grow up thinking this was how a man should treat his wife. Not wanting my daughter to grow up witnessing this abusive marriage as normal gave me enough strength and courage to get an attorney and start the process of getting out.

From the time I decided I needed to get out to the time the divorce was final, it seemed to happen so fast. God aligned everything to work out for me to make it on my own as a 23-year-old mother with a 3-year-old. I know, without a doubt, looking back, that God had rescued me again. He heard my prayers, but He had a different plan for me than what I thought I wanted or needed.

God not saving my marriage would be one of my biggest blessings. In the moment, it seemed like the most devasting failure of my life. Throughout the process, I asked myself so many questions. How did I end up just like my parents so quickly? Why couldn't I make Max happy? What was wrong with me? Why did he cheat on me and physically and verbally abuse me?

The reality was I was dealing with a narcissist, and nothing I did or didn't do could change that. God blessed me by not answering my prayers to save my marriage. He had my godly mate for me, and Max was not him. Unfortunately, I would marry two more times before I would end up with the man God had for me. Yes, you read right! I picked the wrong guy two more times.

MARRIAGE NUMBER 2 ENDED AS QUICKLY AS IT BEGAN

Have you ever gotten through a storm, saw a glimmer of hope, and knew this time would be different? How could you possibly make the same mistake twice? You knew what to look for this time. You would do the opposite of what you did before. There's no way you are going back to an abusive situation again. Does any of this sound familiar to you?

If you said yes, my friend, you are not alone. I had it all figured out. I didn't need any time alone or counseling. I had this relationship thing figured out. Surely, the next guy I would end up with would be the one God had in mind for me. After all, I had been praying, without ceasing, that God would bring the right man into my and my daughter's life.

I was almost 24 years old, and my daughter was three by the time my and Max's divorce was final. I was a full-time personal trainer and group fitness instructor at a popular gym, and I had a lot of amazing and dedicated clients. I was going to be able to make it on my own financially. This was huge because being unable to support my daughter and me alone was one of my biggest fears and why I did not leave my abusive marriage sooner.

I was young, fit, and very attractive. I had never really been single before, so that was uncomfortable. I still had all my same emotional baggage and trauma. Healing and therapy had not occurred before Adam came into my life. He was five years older than me, and it didn't take long for me to latch onto him once he started showing interest in me.

Have you ever experienced a relationship you just wanted to pretend never happened? It was so bad that it felt like a nightmare you wanted to wake up from. That is how I feel about this relationship. I have blacked out most of my memories of Adam and our time together. In this situation, we were two very broken people who had no business being in a relationship, much less with each other.

Adam had recently lost a girlfriend who had been tragically killed in an automobile accident. I had no idea he was still grieving from that and having some mental health issues that he hid very well initially. In his defense, I was such a mess and scared to be alone. I probably wouldn't have cared about these red flags had I noticed them. I was still in the mentality of thinking I could fix people. I saw him for what he could be, not who he was. Have you ever done that with people you loved?

We both drank a lot, and we often took prescription pills to change how we felt. This led to some violent fights. We were in a love tug of war. We'd be madly in love (lust), then suddenly, he'd be breaking up with me telling me what a whore I was. Here we go again. I was a worthless piece of crap to someone else that I thought loved me.

One day, he'd be obsessed with me; the next, he'd tell me he did not want me and how miserable I made him. The I love you; I hate you was emotionally draining. I cried all the time. I had panic attacks regularly. How could this be happening again?

We dated off and on for about nine months. At one point, Adam and Max joined forces to ensure I knew how much of a crazy slut I was. I wanted to die and for the pain to be over at that point. I didn't think I could possibly survive any more abuse. They had convinced me I was completely worthless and no good for anyone.

I finally got enough confidence to break up with Adam for good. I was done. No matter how afraid I was of being alone, I couldn't stay in this relationship any longer. God had placed some amazing spiritual mentors into my life who were leading me through the bible and praying with me and for me. I could do this. I had to do this for me and my daughter.

I was done. I told Adam I wanted to end our relationship. I thought that would be it. Considering how horrible he always told me I was, why would he want to be with me? Breaking up with him turned out to not be that easy. My not wanting him anymore made him want me even more. He was not going to let go of me that easily.

To my surprise, Adam begged me to marry him. He bought me a very expensive ring, and he cried and told me how much he loved me and he how he couldn't live without me. Narcissists are extremely good at making you forget about all the bad they have done. They can suck you back in with a few tears and say, I'm sorry.

I had zero self-worth, fear of abandonment, and fear of making it alone. I was destined to say yes. I didn't have a chance. We were married and off to Mexico for our honeymoon a few weeks after the proposal. We ended up drunk and fighting most of the trip.

Shortly after we got married, he left me. At the same time, I found out I was pregnant. When I told him about the baby, he was so angry. He told me that if I didn't have an abortion, he would make my life hell and never have anything to do with the baby. All I remember after that was falling to the floor crying hysterically, begging him not to leave me.

Sadly, but also for the best, I think, I had a miscarriage. Adam was relieved not to have to worry about that problem anymore. We would end up going through with the divorce, and I would have to pick myself up again after having my heart ripped out one more time.

Surely, I would never make this mistake again. I will get it right next time. I knew what I wanted and didn't want, I thought. I was almost 25 years old, already divorced twice, and a single mother to a little girl who was being raised during toxic and abusive relationships. What was I doing so wrong to deserve this? Why was all this happening to me? I lived in the drama triangle, a complete self-pity and victim mindset.

The cycle of picking the wrong guy and attracting unhealthy guys would continue again. I knew God had someone for me. I knew my godly mate was out there, but I couldn't seem to find him because I was in the wrong mindset and looking in all the wrong places.

ON TO MARRIAGE NUMBER THREE

Have you ever just known without a doubt this was the one? Your heart told you this was the person you should spend the rest of your life with. You could feel it with your whole body. This was the glimmer of hope you were looking for. You knew love still existed, so you dove in headfirst and in a hurry. Never mind looking for red flags. You wouldn't make the same mistake again. There was no way!

The problem with all of that is feelings are indicators, not dictators. Our feelings can lie to us, and we see only what we want to see. We are easily blinded by the desperation and longing in our souls to connect with someone and have them love us unconditionally so that nothing else matters. The desire is so strong, and consuming all the red flags go unnoticed because we don't want to see them.

This was the case going into my next relationship. I had convinced myself that I was in control this time. I would call the shots. I would not be taken advantage of anymore. If healing has not occurred, you cannot jump into another relationship. It is too risky. You are not ready. Trust me.

I was a beautiful, young, very successful personal trainer in my mid-twenties. I had finally gotten some confidence back. Things seemed to be going great for me personally and financially. I made it very clear to any guy that was interested in me that I was in charge. I didn't need them. I would hurt them before I let them hurt me. I went at dating these men like it was a game.

Clearly, I went from one extreme to the other after my second divorce. I had not processed my emotions, forgiven the men who hurt me, or received any kind of therapy. I began going out more to bars when I didn't have my daughter. Men would throw themselves at me, so I used them for free drinks and casual sex. I would make them fall for me, and then I would break it off with them. I had convinced myself this was okay and that I would hurt them before they could hurt me.

Things didn't go as planned. My plan ended up backfiring on me. My relationship with my third husband started out as a bet. You heard me right; I married someone after betting with a friend I could get his cousin to fall for me. It seemed like a fun game then, and I was certain I would win. I won all alright, but as you'd imagine, a relationship that started out as a bet was not exactly godly and stable.

I was at a bar talking with one of my guy friends about his cousin, who was also there. He told me that all the girls fell for his cousin. It was game on after I heard that. I could get him to fall for me. I had fooled myself into thinking I had no problem controlling any situation involving a man. This was going to be easy.

Fast forward… I got Nick, who was fifteen years older than me, to quickly fall in love with me by playing hard to get with an "I don't care I am using you" attitude. Apparently, guys are attracted to that, but I warn you: I do not recommend this approach. The tables turned very quickly as my old behaviors, insecurities, and victim mindset set in after about a month into our relationship.

Taking responsibility for my part in every situation and volatile relationship has been very important in my healing process. We are all broken people with some sort of trauma that we have experienced at one point or another in our lives. For some of us, that trauma is a capital "T," and for some of us, trauma is a little t. It looks different for everyone, but the point is we have all gone through something that causes us to react in unhealthy ways at times.

Nick had gone through a lot in his past, and neither one of us was healthy enough emotionally to be in a relationship that quickly turned into a marriage after about five months of dating. I found out I was pregnant two weeks after we married.

I was certain having a baby with him would mean we'd be together forever.

This time, I had picked someone that was non-confrontational and very passive-aggressive. I was used to fights that involved a lot of confrontation, including yelling and violence. Nick was not going to play that game with me. Whenever I would freak out on him, he would normally leave or say whatever he had to pacify me at the moment. I am sure this was exhausting and emotionally taxing on him. Chaos was my normal, and I took it into our marriage.

After our son was born in December of 2006, I became obsessed with my weight, exercise, and work. I was a full-time personal trainer with an image to uphold. I had to get the weight off fast, especially since I had started training clients again about four weeks after my son was born. Prescription diet pills became my best friend and my energy source to help me feel like a superwoman. I was trying to be the man and the woman of the house, so I needed unlimited energy to fuel my insanity and unrealistic expectations of myself.

Nick never directly called me out on my self-destruction. I did not know how to read between the lines when it came to someone not being happy with me or my behavior. I am sure I ignored every sign of me destroying myself and all my relationships. My prescription diet pill use became dangerously worse very quickly. I was up to needing three to four pills a day, followed by binge drinking to take the edge off and help me go to sleep.

There were a lot of events that led up to the end of our marriage, but I will start with the first set of divorce papers I received a couple of years after we got married. I say first set because, in that last year of marriage, there were three sets of divorce papers by the time we finally ended it for good. For someone with a huge fear of abandonment, this almost killed me. God had a better plan for me, but I didn't know it yet. I was a warrior. I would get through this storm, too.

Have you ever been so caught up in your head and just trying to survive the best way you knew how, and you missed everything telling you that you needed to get yourself together because you were about to lose everything if you didn't? I was so caught up in trying to be what I thought was perfect, doing everything for everyone while trying to uphold this perfect image. I didn't know what hit me when I went to work one day and got served divorce papers saying I could not see my son and could not return to my house.

I fell to the floor sobbing after I received the papers. I was being accused of using drugs and being a danger to my child. The irony was that I honestly had no idea this was coming. I knew I was spiraling out of control with my mental health and addiction to prescription pills and alcohol, but how did this happen without me knowing? Nick even had sex with me the night before he served me divorce papers and kissed me goodbye that morning. We weren't even in a fight.

I get it together quickly whenever my back is against the wall. I got sober immediately and got an attorney. I sought help through AA and showed Nick I could be the woman he needed me to be. After a few months, he wanted me back. The divorce papers were gone. I had a feeling of relief and hope that this marriage could be saved. I thought Everything would be okay if I could be exactly who he wanted me to be.

It didn't take long for Nick to get upset with me again and leave. This time, I would file divorce papers on him. I was still sober. I didn't feel like I had done anything wrong. Why did he keep leaving me? I was sincerely clueless as to what I was doing to upset him. I am sure he had plenty of valid reasons, but I didn't know what they were because there was zero communication in our marriage or any type of healthy conflict. I am sure he was fearful to share his true feelings with me because I normally freaked out and got defensive if I felt like my character was being attacked.

It didn't take long for him to want me back again when he saw that I was moving on. The second set of divorce papers would be dropped. I had hope again. Surely, this time it was going to work out. He wanted me back. Why in the world would he leave me again?

I got comfortable and let my guard down on our relationship, my mental health, and my disease of addiction. I was in full-blown relapse mode shortly after we reconciled for the second time. I was still personal training at this time and trying to maintain the superwoman status. If I could just do enough things for Nick, my kids, and my clients, everyone would be happy with me. If I could just perform high enough, no one would leave or be mad at me. I needed extra energy to do everything I was trying to do for approval. Prescription pills were the answer to getting the massive energy I needed.

Even though Nick would participate in drinking alcohol with me, it didn't take him long to bail on me for a third time. Nick was partying with me. I didn't think he would accuse me of endangering my children and have everything taken away from me again. How could he if he was doing it with me? Oh, he figured it out. I completely got set up and blind-sided this third and final time.

I did not get served divorce papers, but he told me that I would lose everything if I didn't check myself in somewhere to get help for my addiction. All I had to do was get help, and I would get my family back. He didn't have to tell me twice. I would do whatever it took to get my family back.

I checked myself into a dual-diagnosis mental health/addiction hospital where I sought help for as long as they would keep me. It was not glamorous at all. It was a state-run mental hospital where they basically got you detoxed, treated your mental health issues with some prescription medications, and sent you on your way.

FROM THE MENTAL HOSPITAL TO REHAB

One of the most devasting days of my life that became a blessing in disguise happened on the third day I was at the mental hospital. I thought my husband was coming to see me for a visitation, but instead, I was greeted by a stranger who figured out how to get into a private facility and serve me my third set of divorce papers in less than two years. I fell to the ground, sobbing uncontrollably. I could not do anything to defend myself. I was going to lose everything. The promise of returning to my family was ripped away from me in moments.

I feel like I need to share a little more about this marriage and time in my life because so many defining moments happened. It was also a time in my life when I was in full-blown victim mode. I felt like life was happening to me and not for me. I blamed everyone and everything other than myself for the position I was in. This mentality blinded me, paralyzed me, and kept me from taking responsibility for my part, which would propel me out of the drama triangle I was trapped in.

Granted, a lot was happening to me and had happened to me. I was clearly a victim of people and my circumstances. I have only shared a small portion of what I have gone through up to this point. Have you ever felt so victimized that you could not see past the pain you were going through? Have you felt like your heart was physically broken and being ripped out of your chest? Every step and breath you took consumed all the energy you had left in your body. Have you ever felt like you were merely surviving and wished you could just go to sleep and not wake up?

If you have experienced any of this, you are not alone, my friend. I lived like this for decades. I am here to share my experience in this mental prison, so you no longer feel alone. As you keep reading, I pray I give you hope and tools that allow you to break out of the prison you have been living in for far too long. I am living proof that there is another side and another way that you can find joy, peace, and self-worth no matter what is happening around you that is out of your control.

God has placed many earth angels in my life at just the right time. I don't remember the name of the nurse who comforted me the day I got the third set of divorce papers, but I do remember she played an important part in speaking the truth into me and encouraging me to seek further in-patient help.

I will share more about my time in treatment in the next chapter. Just know that I thought I was taking drastic measures to do whatever I needed to do to get my family back and for my husband not to go through with the divorce. God had a very different plan for me. While I felt like I was dying from a broken heart, God was preparing my true godly mate for me.

HOW I STOPPED LETTING MY ANGER AND RESENTMENT FOR THESE MEN CONSUME ME

I am now a health, fitness, and mindset coach. God has allowed me to use my pain as my purpose to help others truly. I am beyond grateful for everything that I have gone through because it allows me to empathize with my clients on a deeper level. I can meet them where they are, and most of the time, I know exactly how they are feeling because I have experienced and overcome what they are currently going through.

One day, I was doing a mindset coaching session with one of my clients who was having difficulty letting her resentment for her abusive, narcissistic ex-husband consume her. She was allowing her anger and resentment toward him to take over, leading to her self-sabotaging her health journey. She desperately wanted these feelings to go away because she knew they were hurting her more than they were hurting her ex, and it was holding her back from leveling up in her health journey.

Have you ever been in this place where your anger for someone who has hurt you continues to destroy you daily because you can't let it go? Do you feel like your abuser is still abusing you even though you left them long ago? Forgiveness and letting go are tricky, but if you can be open to thinking differently, there is freedom on the other side of forgiveness.

When my client asked me how I could move on and not let my anger for these men that had hurt me consume me, I had to think about it. How did I move on? What steps led me to freedom from an all-consuming resentment that I felt in my body and caused me to self-sabotage myself and my relationships constantly?

First, forgiveness had taken a lot of time and intentionality and prayer, lots of prayer. I prayed for them. Ephesians 4:32 says, "Be kind and compassionate to one another, forgiving each other, just as in Christ God forgave you." This is easier said than done! Why would I want to forgive someone who hurt me so badly? Why do they deserve to be forgiven? How could I possibly let them off the hook? I believe in God, and I want to obey him. If the Bible says we need to forgive, then I am going to trust God and that He has what is best for me in mind by telling me to forgive others as He has forgiven me.

I explained to my teary-eyed client how I began this process of forgiveness when I did not feel like it or mean it when I prayed about it. I trusted that if I prayed for my exes and told God that I forgave them, the feelings would eventually come. It was for me to heal. I was not letting them off the hook, but I had to see them with compassion to heal.

They are broken people just like me. They have their own trauma that has happened to them, and unfortunately, they had allowed that trauma to trigger toxic reactions that spilled into our relationship. They had not healed from what had been done to them or was happening to them while we were together. My heart softened toward them. It wasn't about me. I just happened to be the one they took their pain out on. I also took my unresolved pain from my childhood out on them too.

If I am honest, the brokenness in me that led me to act crazy and emotional probably triggered a lot of old traumas in them. Two broken people can really bring out the worst in each other. It is so sad, and I see it happening with so many of my clients' relationships. They are constantly trying to figure out how to fix their partner when the answer lies in fixing themselves and modeling the behavior, they want their partner to give them.

I had to get outside of myself and stop making their abusive behavior all about me. By doing this, I could release them into God's hands and regain my power. They hurt people. Hurt people hurt people. I felt sorry for them, which helped me feel sincere when I prayed for their salvation, healing, and prosperity.

How did I know that what I was doing was really working? I could test this theory the day I had this eye-opening conversation with my client. I went to an awards program for one of my kids that evening, where I would see his dad for the first time in about a year. If I felt the anger and resentment in my body when I was in the same room with him, I would know that I had not truly forgiven him and let it go. This was going to be the test.

I was happy to report to my client that I didn't feel triggered in my body or experience any anxiety when I stood beside him after the program was over. It may have taken many years of consistently praying and choosing to look at him through compassionate eyes, but it worked. I was free from resentment. I had my power back. It can work for you, too, if you are consistent in your efforts to see the person who hurt you as a broken person just like you and you are open to thinking differently.

CHAPTER EIGHT

THE PILLS NO LONGER MADE ME SUPERWOMAN!

"MOTHER'S LITTLE HELPER"

It did not take me long to find an article about prescription stimulant abuse in moms and the dangers that come with it. According to www.drugrehab.us, "Mother's little helper" has been used for decades. In 1966, The Rolling Stones released a hit song about the abuse of drugs, like Valium, by mothers looking to take the edge off a busy day. Now, some moms are using different substances to get through the day:

prescription stimulants. Although they can boost much-desired energy, many women develop a drug addiction to these commonly prescribed "legitimate" medications."

The article entitled "Mother's Little Helper- Prescription Stimulant Abuse in Moms.... And the Dangers," found at *www.drugrehab.us* describes why moms are abusing stimulants describes me perfectly and why I needed massive amounts of energy to perform like the superwoman I thought I had to be for the love and approval I longed for. Have you ever felt like you had so much to do but not enough energy to do it all? Have you felt like you were so exhausted before the day even started, and just the normal everyday tasks of working, being a mom, and a wife were weighing you down, and you just wanted to crawl back into bed and binge-watch TV or simply check out? You are not alone.

The article states, "The demands placed on mothers in this culture can feel overwhelming. From single moms to homeschooling moms to moms who work outside the home, many feel pressured to be the master multitasker. Some mothers turn to stimulants to help them focus better on their responsibilities or help them make it through a hectic day." This was me. I thought I had to do it all and do it perfectly. My self-worth was wrapped up in how much I could get done and getting praised by others for how awesome I was doing everything.

Not only did the pills give me energy, but they also suppressed my appetite. I constantly felt fat and uncomfortable in my skin. It was a win if I could use the pills to get energy and not eat, which would make me feel skinny! I was a very busy personal trainer. If I weren't eating throughout the day, the prescription diet pills, pain pills, and ADHD medications would help me have killer workouts and give me the energy to train my clients and care for my family. The pills were like magic to me. They were the solution to my excessive need for energy. A doctor prescribed them. That must mean they were safe.

MY PRESCRIPTION PILL USE STARTED INNOCENTLY

After my first divorce, I was in my early 20s, a personal trainer and group fitness instructor, and a mom of a 3-year-old. I was scared that I wouldn't be able to make it on my own. God had rescued me from a very abusive relationship, but now I had to figure out how I would be successful enough to support myself and my little girl. Personal training was no longer extra income. It was my sole income. I had to step up my game and build up my clientele.

It all started so innocently. I learned about prescription diet pills from people at my gym who were getting them off the internet. If they were using them, surely, they were safe. Remember, I was someone with an extremely addictive personality. One of anything was never enough to satisfy me.

Looking back, it all seems so crazy that you could get prescription strength diet pills off the internet. They were highly addictive, and no one worried about the long-term effects. It was a quick fix, and everyone loves instant gratification.

I took them as prescribed for a long time. There were a couple of problems that surfaced quickly, though. The diet pills made me want to smoke cigarettes, and very on edge and irritable. I also needed to drink alcohol at the end of the day to take the edge off and go to sleep. I would go all day without eating, then binge eat at night before bed when the pills wore off.

I was hooked instantly. I did not see anything wrong with what I was doing. I justified and rationalized my using them by telling myself everyone was doing it. I was being super productive and helping so many people get fit while being a young single mother. I had no intention of stopping any time soon.

I went to bed thinking about how I would feel when I got up the next morning and how I would immediately pop that pill in my mouth as soon as I got out of bed. I got a euphoric feeling and a slight burst of energy just thinking about taking the pill. I craved them and obsessed with them. I also feared running out before I could get my hands on more. I was officially addicted and could not live without my "little helper."

I WAS LIVING AS A VICTIM OF MY ENVIRONMENT

It became a little harder and expensive to maintain my diet pill use. After a couple of years, I built a tolerance, which was not enough to do the job anymore. I quickly realized I could get the same effect the diet pills gave me by taking prescription pain pills, cough medicine, and ADHD medication. They all gave me a euphoric high and unstoppable energy. I felt amazing when I took them. My obsession consumed me. I would do whatever I had to do to get my hands on pills even if that meant spending a ton of money, stealing them from other people, and doctor shopping.

Have you ever felt like you were living an out-of-body experience where you had lost all control? Instead of you having control, everything outside you had control over you and how you would react. Have your emotions and how you will go about your day been controlled by your partner/spouse, work, your children, the substance you are addicted to that is getting you through your day, friends, or even co-workers? If you said yes to any of these, you, my friend, are living as a victim to your environment like I did most of my life.

Where you place your energy is where you place your attention. Sadly, we are addicted to the emotions of the past. We will unconsciously look for ways to find those emotions from the past because we are comfortable being in victim mode. This is how most people stay stuck. It isn't on purpose. It is how we are hard-wired.

I was on a perpetual loop, living as a victim of my environment. Looking back, I see that I was using anything that would give me energy (mostly prescription drugs) to rescue myself and be the hero of my story. If I performed at a high, very unrealistic level, I had enough self-worth to keep my head above water.

I had convinced myself that I wasn't doing anything wrong by taking pills. Nobody was getting hurt. In fact, I was able to take care of everyone better. The people that I would steal pills from didn't need them. They had full prescription bottles that had been sitting in their medicine cabinets for a very long time. This was my insanity and addiction talking. Justifying and rationalizing behavior is typical among addicts.

90 DAYS IN TREATMENT

I mentioned earlier it was a miracle from God that I could go to an amazing treatment center against my family's wishes. They all thought I should just get it together and return home to care for everything like they were used to me doing. I knew I needed help in a controlled environment. I had to do whatever it took to get my family back.

Going to treatment was the right decision, but as I knew it, my entire world fell apart while I was away. Everything I had been begging God to save would not be saved. Sometimes, unanswered prayers can be a blessing from God, but at the time, I felt like I was literally dying inside from the loss.

My husband went from coming to visit me, and he even had sex with me on one visit, to suddenly not answering my or my counselor's calls. I thought I was on the road to save my marriage because I was doing everything he told me to do that would get my family back. Why was this happening to me?

I was still stuck in the mindset that life happened to me. It was torturous. I could not see past the moment. How could I possibly survive being left again? Would I get my children back? How would I make it on my own financially? These thoughts consumed me.

My counselor finally got in touch with Nick. She was trying to plan for family day and my aftercare once I left treatment. Nick told her that it wasn't his problem because he divorced me. You read that right! He divorced me and took everything, even my child, without me knowing it happened. I had absolutely no reason to believe he would go through with the divorce while I was in treatment. How could he even do that without me being present in court?

Once I overcame the shock, I got it together and moved forward with my after-care plans. I wanted to do everything the treatment center suggested. I had to get this right. I was willing to do whatever it took. I would even agree to their recommendation of going to live in a sober living house for a few months after treatment.

Everything started to fall into place for me to move on, or so I thought. Out of nowhere, I would get another life-altering bomb dropped on me. This one came out of nowhere and would change how I looked at myself and my relationship with my mom. This news deserves a chapter of its own. Keep reading!

HE WANTED ME BACK THEN HE LEFT ME AGAIN

When you are in recovery, they tell you to take it "One Day at a Time" and "Do the Next Right Thing," and the miracles will come. Well, I was banking on those promises. When I decide to do something, I am all in, whether it is good or bad. I was going to use my powers for good!

I was shocked when Nick called me late one night and told me he wanted me back. He wanted me to come home and for us to be together. This was the moment I had been waiting for. I had given up and begun to move on; he wanted me back out of nowhere. I packed up my stuff and left the sober living house the next day to return home.

Nick had sold our house while I was gone. He was renting a duplex and had a girl living with him and my 3-year-old son whom we used to party with. I had no idea this was happening while I was away. At that moment, I didn't care what he had done while I was gone. All I cared about was that we were back together, and I wouldn't be alone. Nothing else mattered.

I was moving forward with my recovery. I was working with my sponsor and going to AA meetings regularly. Unfortunately, Nick was still the same person. He had not done anything to work on his recovery as a co-dependent married to an addict. It is more likely than not that where there is an alcoholic, there is a co-dependent attachment to them. A relationship is unlikely to be healthy and working unless both parties recover.

Only a couple of weeks passed before my whole world would be turned upside down again. Nick didn't come home from work and would not answer my phone calls or texts. Devastation consumed me. I had no idea what I had done wrong. Why did he leave me again? I was doing everything I could to be the wife and mom he told me he wanted me to be. I was blindsided again.

The good news was that I still had both of my kids, and he could not accuse me of doing anything bad. I was truly innocent this time. There was no way this was my fault. Once again, I was a victim. Life was happening to me. Life was always happening to me.

My relationship with Nick had officially come to an end. When he finally decided to talk to me, he told me that he could not be the man I needed him to be. We did not fight. He didn't accuse me of anything. A feeling of acceptance finally came over me, and I had to move on with my life. I am beyond grateful that God did not answer my prayers to save my marriage. I did not know it yet, but God had my perfect godly mate ready for me, and I would meet him soon.

MY ADDICTION TO PILLS AND ALCOHOL WOULD CONTINUE TO HAUNT A LITTLE LONGER

Even though I went to an amazing treatment center for 90 days and worked the program of AA for a while afterward, I would not stay sober long. I had not had complete healing from my trauma. In fact, there was more trauma to come. I let the triggers from my PTSD, mental health issues, and victim mentality take over most of the time, and I would always turn to a substance to change how I felt instead of dealing with the emotions head-on.

I did not know how to deal with life on life's terms. I did not know how to process and talk about what was tormenting me inside. I only knew how to stop the pain by numbing it with pills and/or alcohol, avoiding it, and building a fortress around myself for protection.

Here is what I learned. I had built such a thick fortress around myself just to survive my everyday life; nothing and no one could get inside. This fortress not only protected me from the bad, but it also kept out happiness and love. Most days, I put on a good show that I was happy and content, but inside, I was slowly dying.

On the nights when I started drinking heavily again, I would get eaten alive with anger, resentment, self-pity, and fear of what would happen to me next. I would pray to God to let me go to sleep and not wake up. The addiction had become too strong for me to conquer on my own. The fortress was keeping people out who could help me. I was too afraid to let people in because I could not fathom being hurt and abandoned again.

This fortress protected me for a little while, and it felt like a good thing. The problem was that the fortress was so thick and impenetrable that I couldn't let happiness and joy in either. The fortress had become a prison I was trapped in. It was a prison of my own making. Have you ever felt trapped in a prison that you had the keys to but didn't know how to use to unlock the doors?

My prayer for you is to be able to use the keys God has given you to unlock the doors of your self-created prison to not only get out but to thrive as the powerful person He created you to be. I want you to see that there is hope no matter how bad your life has been. You can do the work like I have to free yourself from all that has entrapped you for so long.

WISDOM IN MY SOBRIETY AND HEALING

1. The very thing that discourages you is the very thing that develops you!

2. Pain is the high cost of growth!

3. The only person who will dig you out of your hole is you!

4. We don't lose; we only win or learn! If you can work through your pain, I guarantee you on the other side is a reward.

5. You will find peace when you go to war with yourself. You don't find peace by sitting there, binge-watching TV shows, scrolling social media, or staying in bed doing nothing. When you start challenging yourself at every turn, breaking down barriers, and getting back up, you will find peace at the end of that!

6. We all have our own tests and traumas, whether it be addiction, abuse, eating disorders, depression, anxiety, insecurity, or any other paralyzing issue you are struggling to overcome. The only way to overcome it is for you and you alone to face it.

7. You must do your best work when you are least motivated and when you don't feel like doing it. You've

got to make yourself get up and do the hard things anyway and challenge yourself.

8. Try to be 1% better than you were last week.

9. When you are casual about like, you become a casualty.

10. "Don't say I am having a bad day. Instead, say I am having a character-building day." (Les Brown)

CHAPTER NINE

I WASN'T WHO I THOUGHT I WAS!

WHAT IF THE OPPOSITE IS TRUE?

Have you ever felt in your gut that something wasn't right? Have you ever had an intuition that you weren't being told everything? Secrets were being kept from you, but you just couldn't put your finger on it. Your mind goes all over the place, fantasizing about what the secret could possibly be. Our imaginations can run wild with the stories we tell ourselves in this scenario.

At our house, we have implemented a tool to help us not go to the worst-case scenario. I want to encourage you to put this into practice at your house, yourself, and the whole family. If you find your mind going to a dark place when you don't know all the facts about a situation or person, ask yourself, "What if the opposite were true?". Almost every time, the opposite of the story we tell ourselves about something or someone is true. What we are catastrophizing about is far from reality because we don't know the facts. We will make up a story in our heads with the worst possible outcome in an attempt to protect ourselves.

If we think we know what is coming, it is easier to go ahead and get in defense mode. We are ready for whatever we are assuming is coming our way. Here is an example. Say you text a close friend, and she doesn't respond immediately like she normally does. Immediately, you start thinking that she is mad at you. You do a replay of the last time you talked to try and figure out what you could have possibly done to upset her. You assume the absolute worst. You didn't do anything wrong, but you are sure she is mad at you about something.

Stop at that moment. Take a breath. Ground yourself in the present moment, and then ask yourself out loud, "What if the opposite were true?'. What is the opposite? Maybe she didn't see your text. Maybe she opened the text, got distracted, and then forgot to respond. Maybe she is going through something painful that had absolutely nothing to do with you, and she doesn't have the capacity to respond.

In most cases, the opposite is true. Stop assuming things. The worst is not always what is happening. I realize if you have lived a life of trauma, it can feel like your reality is always the worst-case scenario. The Bible says in Philippians 4:8, "And now, dear brothers and sisters, one final thing. Fix your thoughts on what is true, honorable, right, pure, lovely, and admirable. Think about these things that are all worthy of praise."

What you focus on grows. If we are always focusing on the worst, we will more likely than not find what we are looking for with evidence to support it. You have the power to flip the narrative. Asking yourself, "What if the opposite were true?" is a great starting place to practice flipping the narrative to come out of a victim mentality.

UNFORTUNATELY, IN THIS INSTANCE, THE OPPOSITE WAS NOT TRUE, FOR ME

For as long as I can remember, I always felt like something was off. I could never put my finger on it, and my mind would go all over the place trying to figure out why my mom kept me at arm's length. What did I do wrong? Why didn't she act like she wanted to be around me or love me? Where did this disconnect come from?

All the crazy things I was thinking were far from the truth. So, I guess the opposite was true in a sense, but it was not in a positive way. It was something that had never crossed my mind. After I found out what the secret was that my parents were keeping from me, so many things made sense, looking back on different events in my life.

One moment traumatized me and broke my heart for a very long time. My mom could have taken this opportunity to tell me the truth, but she didn't. I am sure she had her reasons. Maybe she froze and couldn't get the words out that day I told her that a very close family member had raped me at age 23.

We were standing in the office of one of the counselors at the mental hospital I had checked myself into before I went to treatment. He encouraged me to open up to my mom. I shared a deep, dark secret that had been tormenting me for several years at that point in my life. Hysterically crying, I blurted out what had happened to me, and all my mom could say was, "I don't know what part you had in it.". I cannot tell you how many times I have played this day over and over in my head. I questioned my validity and whether he did rape me.

If you are a survivor of sexual abuse, have you ever felt like it was your fault? Have you ever felt like maybe you were asking for it? I had been extremely close with this family member my entire life. I trusted him. I had been drinking heavily the night it happened. So maybe it was my fault. After a lot of therapy, I understand it was not my fault, but I blame myself for drinking too much and blacking out the night it happened.

Why didn't my mom take that opportunity to tell me the truth about where I came from and who I was? That is not my story to tell. I must believe she didn't mean to hurt me. My mom has experienced her own trauma, which probably has much to do with why she held on to this secret for as long as possible.

The day I finally found out, I was sitting in my counselor's office with my aunt and uncle, who financially supported me after I got out of treatment. Once again, another counselor encouraged me to share what had happened to me with my family members. My dad had died a year before, and I was extremely blessed to have the support of my dad's brother and his wife. It was a God thing because I was not close with them at all before all of this. I had prayed for a miracle, and God brought them into my life for support.

I know you are dying to know what the secret is. Well, here you go! Full of fear and anxiety, I could hardly get the words out about the family member raping me, but I told them. Right after I told them, my uncle looked at my aunt in a way I will never forget. He then turned to me and said sadly, "Your dad wasn't your real dad.". Here we go again. What in the world! Why did he feel the need to share this life-shattering news with me now?

I guess he thought the idea of the family member raping me wouldn't be as bad if I knew this family member wasn't my family member. I felt like what I was telling them was being minimized, and at the same time, the reality was setting in that my entire life, I wasn't who I thought I was. It was like finding out I was adopted. The trauma of this news would lead me to many more years of substance abuse to cope with the feelings of all of this.

I AM A DONOR BABY

An anonymous sperm donor from a sperm bank conceived me. Most people would think that this is a blessing. Many people have said, "Your mom and dad wanted you so badly that they took extreme measures to have you." I did not feel these warm and fuzzy feelings. I was angry and resentful that I had been lied to my entire life, and to top it all off, my mom let me think a family member raped me and that I had something to do with it.

I had always felt like I was a burden to my parents. I was left home alone or with babysitters all the time. I did not feel an emotional unconditional love from my parents. I had always felt like my dad looked at me like a sexual object. Now I knew why.

Finding out at the age of 29 in a counseling session where I was opening up about rape was not the most ideal way to find out your dad was not your real dad. In any case, it was the hand I was dealt. I had to figure out how to move forward without letting all the negative feelings overtake me and lead me to a perpetual self-sabotage.

Sadly, I let the anger, betrayal, and resentment of the news overtake me for about ten years. Every time I looked in the mirror, I saw something different. Questions flooded my mind. Who was the donor? What did he look like? What was my family origin? Why was I so fit and muscular when my mom hated exercise? Did I have any siblings? I could go on and on.

I would get drunk and go down a rabbit hole of emotions and questions that didn't serve me. I kept myself in a victim mindset. I was angry at my parents for lying to me my entire life. I was angry at the donor for giving his sperm away to create a child. He would not know whether they were going to a loving or neglectful home. The anger and resentment consumed me often. I didn't know how to let it go and move on. I needed answers.

STATISTICS ABOUT SPERM-DONOR KIDS

I found these statistics very interesting and extremely accurate in my case. There are so many of us out there. I was conceived in 1980 when the procedure was new. The first Cryobank opened in the United States in the early 1970s. They were largely run by men and offered frozen sperm from anonymous donors (often college students) to mostly infertile couples.

My parents used a donor because my dad had a vasectomy before he married my mom. I was told that he tried to reverse it, but that didn't work. My parents first investigated adoption and heard about using a sperm donor. My mom was 22 years younger than my dad and his third wife. My mom wanted to have a baby with him.

My mom wanted to keep this secret from me forever, so she has not given me many details. It has only been occasional awkward conversations with very few answers. She said they went in for the procedure, and it took the first time. That was that. It worked, and it was never to be talked about again.

People in my age group, born in the late 70s to 80s, who were conceived by an anonymous sperm donor from a Cryobank aren't really talked about. The reality is that most of us are not okay. Our parents were told by the doctors not to tell us the truth and to pretend like it never happened.

According to an article entitled, *The Sperm-Donor Kids Are Not Really All Right*, on *slate.com*, "Each year, an estimated 30,000-60,000 children are born in this country via artificial insemination, but the number is only an educated guess. Neither the fertility industry nor any other entity must report on the statistics."

The article says, "While adoption is often the center of controversy, it turns out that sperm donation raises many different but equally complex and sometimes troubling issues. Two-thirds of adult donor offspring agree with the statement, "My sperm donor is half of who I am." Nearly half are disturbed that money was involved in their conception. More than half say that when they see someone who resembles them, they wonder if they are related. About two-thirds affirm the right of donor offspring to know the truth about their origins.

Regardless of socioeconomic status, donor offspring are twice as likely as those raised by biological parents to report problems with the law before age 25. They are more than twice as likely to report having struggled with substance abuse. And they are about 1.5 times as likely to report depression or other mental health problems."

I agree with the article about donor offspring suffering more than adopted ones. "...hurting more, feeling more confused, and feeling more isolated from their families. The donor offspring are more likely than the adopted to have struggled with addiction and delinquency, and, like the adopted, a significant number have confronted depression or other mental illnesses. Nearly half of the donor offspring and more than half of adoptees agree, "It is better to adopt than to use donated sperm or eggs to have a child."

I feel in my heart what Lynne Spencer, a nurse, and donor-conceived adult, says so eloquently, "When you grow up, and your instincts are telling you one thing, and your parents, the people you are supposed to be able to trust the most in your life are telling you something else, your whole sense of what is true and not true is all confused."

MY DONOR SIBLINGS AND I WERE NOT OKAY

How do I know donor-conceived people in my age group are not okay? Well, I thought it would be a good idea to submit my DNA to a website to see if I could figure out more about where I came from. I wasn't necessarily looking for my biological father or even family, for that matter. I was looking for health history and family origin. I was tired of looking at myself in the mirror and seeing something different every time. I wanted answers.

I found out some health history and some family origin and way more than what I bargained for. I would be hit with another ton of bricks that would give me more reason to stay a victim, be depressed, and then drink over it. Here we go again.

To my surprise, which is an understatement, I kept matching with more and more half-siblings over time. As far as I know, I have about 20 half-siblings with the same donor as me. It seemed like every time I logged into the site, I would get notified of a new relative. They are from all over and all about the same age as me. I was born in 1981. Out of all the donor siblings I matched with, I was one of the few who knew my dad wasn't my real dad. Most of them found out after submitting their DNA to the website for other reasons.

We were shocked and full of mixed emotions as we found each other and connected. I was dying to have a family connection. I fantasized about connecting with my long-lost family like you see on 20/20 or Dateline. My fantasy would turn into a nightmare quickly.

Most of my newfound siblings were just discovering that their parents had lied to them their entire lives. They were going through all the emotions of being lied to and betrayed. I'm assuming it's kind of like finding out you were adopted. It is a feeling I can only describe as having your heart ripped out and being hit over the head with a two-by-four. It hurts. It hurts bad.

I had about four years to process. I was ready to connect, and most of them were not. I was also back in my addiction and mental health struggles. Looking back, I am sure they thought I was crazy. I met one of my sisters right away. She is a beautiful and talented actress and model in Las Vegas. We connected, but my expectations were just too much. I longed for a sister. She just wanted a friend.

I got tired of getting my feelings hurt, and the feelings of rejection became too much very quickly. It was not anyone's fault. I was too needy. I was back in my addiction, which had me very irrational. I wanted something they did not have the capacity to give yet, or maybe ever. None of us were okay, really.

I ended up blocking all of them in my contacts and on Facebook because every time I saw them on social media, it reminded me of what I would never have. Jealousy and rejection consumed me. I had to move on because it was taking me down fast.

We found the donor's sister, which led to us finding out who the donor was. He denied that he was our donor, and understandably, he didn't want to have anything to do with us. Why would he? He was just donating sperm to get through medical school. No strings attached. He did not sign up to be a father to God knows how many kids. There are a lot of us.

I HAD TO MOVE ON

I had to get out of this torture I was putting myself through. The only way I knew how to do this was to detach from all of them and stop trying altogether. In haste and anger, I unfriended and blocked all of them on social media and my phone contacts. I would leave them before they could leave me. This was becoming my pattern and how I protected myself from abandonment and rejection.

I built a fortress around myself for protection. It was a good thing for a little while. The problem was I stopped coming out of the fortress altogether or letting people in. I was blocking out the bad, and at the same time, I was also blocking out all the good in my life. The fortress became a prison I would battle daily to get out of for several more years.

Almost a year later, God brought a gift I never expected into my life. It was a gift that would bring me a healthy body and a community that would become better than any blood family that I could imagine.

This gift of health began my healing process. I signed up for a diet to lose 10 pounds and gain more energy. I was an overweight personal trainer stuck in the trap of trying to work off a bad diet. I worked out like I had since I was 20 years old, two hours a day, five to six days a week, at extremely high intensities. My workout wasn't working anymore. I was desperately searching for something to help me feel better and lose weight that didn't include diet pills or starving myself. I was miserable and living a meh life.

God had blessed me with so much more than losing ten pounds and gaining energy! My new habits were so much more than a diet! It was a health journey. I lost 43 pounds in 3.5 months, started sleeping through the night without sleeping pills, got off some of my medications, got my joy and energy back, and so much more.

I signed up to coach this amazing plan and pay this gift forward. Everyone needed what I had, and I was on a mission to help as many people as possible that God allowed to become the best version of themselves. I had a new purpose and drive in me that was unstoppable. In my first 3.5 years of health coaching, I helped over 1,000 people get healthy. I shifted from selfishness and self-pity to passionately serving others.

The other coaches in my new health community quickly became my new family. My clients also became like family to me. I cared about them deeply. My heart was beginning to open, but I still had work to do. Honestly, I still battle daily to let the walls of my fortress down to let people in to experience love and connection in a new, healthy way.

I would like to tell you that all my problems were solved by getting healthy and coaching, but they were not yet. The key word there is yet! God continued to open doors for opportunity, growth, healing, and becoming the woman He created me to be. It was up to me to walk through the doors and trust Him.

Do you ever resist God and the doors He opens for you? Do you want to go through them but can't because fear paralyzes you and holds you back? You know deep down that if you just take a chance, rip the Band-Aid® off, and do it scared, miracles are possible on the other side. This is where I want to encourage you to marry the process and divorce the results.

I believe in the old cliché, when one door closes, another door opens, because I have experienced countless doors closing and opening in my life. I never lost my faith in God through all my pain and trauma. I never stopped believing that God is still in the miracle business. I had to believe because not believing in God and His miracles and blessings meant my loss of hope and death.

The family I envisioned was not God's very best for my life. He had something so much better planned. My dreamer was slightly broken while finding "family" and losing them. I released my expectations into God's hands and trusted that He had something more for me. I just needed to stay on His path and pray for Him to keep me in the center of His will, and everything would work out for God's glory! I kept putting one foot in front of the other, focusing on serving others. That is when the magic started happening.

CHAPTER TEN

I FINALLY FOUND MY GODLY MATE!

"God, please bring my godly mate into my life. Let him recognize me, and I recognize him without a doubt!" was my constant prayer for many years. I prayed that prayer without ceasing, just like the Bible says to do. I knew deep down in my heart, amid all the abusive and toxic relationships, my soulmate was out there. How much longer would I have to endure the pain of not being with the one God had for me?

Jamie Kern Lima said, "Rejection is God's protection.". Read that again and again. Write it down as a reminder when you feel like everything is falling apart. This revelation is a game changer. I wish I had heard this quote while going through all my failed marriages, which felt like the ultimate rejection every step of the way.

I also begged God to save my marriage. Have you ever wanted something so bad that you just knew God wanted for you, too? Have you ever begged, pleaded, and bargained with God to reconcile a situation you just knew had to be His will for your life? Why in the world would God allow divorce and abuse to happen? In the moments of crying out to my Savior, none of it made sense when I kept getting left.

Of course, God hates divorce, but in my situation, it was necessary. The gut-wrenching pain I experienced was all part of a bigger plan. I know now that part of that plan is to share my story and give you hope. If you are going through a breakup and feel like your life is over, hang on, pray, and believe. I knew God had someone for me, but I could have never imagined how beautiful a godly marriage could be.

God may or may not restore your marriage or relationship. In my case, divorce had to happen three times. I kept going back to the same toxic relationships over and over. I have often heard that we are addicted to past behaviors and emotions because they are familiar and comfortable. We will always drift back to past behaviors unless we are willing to outlast the temporary pain and discomfort of change and growth.

I was the definition of insanity. I was doing the same things repeatedly, expecting a different result. To stop this insanity, I had to surrender my will and life to God's care. True surrender put me in the center of God's will. I prayed for God to put His perfect plan, will, and purpose into action in my life. I let go and let God, and the miracles began to happen in my life.

God brought my godly mate into my life, and there was no doubt that my husband, Chris, was "the one." Chris tells the story so much better. It is kind of our thing to let him tell our story when we share with others about how we met and ended up getting married after only six weeks of dating. I will do my best to tell our story as well as Chris.

MY FIRST ENCOUNTER WITH CHRIS

Do you believe that everything happens for a reason? Do you believe that God orchestrates encounters with sometimes seemingly random people that will later play a role in your life for one reason or another? I don't call it fate! I call these encounters a "God thing."

The first time I saw my hot husband, Chris, was at a retreat that was a last-ditch effort to save my marriage to Nick. I was desperately doing anything and everything not to get another divorce. My focus was more on saving my marriage and getting Nick to change than working on myself, which I should have been doing while I was at this retreat.

At the retreat, we were split up into two large groups. If you came with someone, you were in separate groups the entire weekend. Being placed in a group separate from their partner allowed the person to focus on working on themselves without distractions. Let's be honest; we can only fix ourselves. I was so focused on fixing my marriage and Nick that I couldn't begin to work on myself even though he was in an entirely different room the whole weekend.

At the time, I was an emotional wreck, and I was secretly taking prescription diet pills to help me "have energy" and engage with everyone. Remember, I wasn't good in large crowds sober. I sabotaged my experience but looking back. It just wasn't my time to get better. I didn't even know how to wrap my mind around the concept of focusing on myself because I was so used to doing and being everything for everyone. You don't have to look in the mirror if you convince yourself you are living a life of total service to others. My time for true self-healing would come years later.

Chris had also come to the retreat to save his marriage without his wife. She refused to come. I had never met Chris before. Have you ever had a first encounter with someone, and you just knew that you had met before but couldn't put your finger on it? Have you ever experienced an immediate connection and energy with a stranger like you have known them forever? My first encounter with Chris was like running into an old friend, but we had never met before.

Chris and I were both at the retreat to save our marriages. We did not flirt or engage with each other in any inappropriate way. He saw me like no one else saw me there. I was not hiding my pain and distraction from him like I was with everyone else. I felt like he truly cared about me and what was happening inside me.

Neither of us could figure out where we knew each other from, but we felt it. He was kind and extremely caring whenever he spoke to me that weekend. I didn't think much about it. I was there to save my marriage and fix Nick. I was not there to flirt or meet someone to hook up with. We went our separate ways, and I never thought I would hear from him or see him again.

Chris was tasked with the title of large group leader. He was in charge of checking on everyone after we left to return home, where we were supposed to use the tools we had received from this life-changing weekend. Sure, I felt the high you get from leaving this kind of experience for a little while. For a moment, I thought my life and marriage were on the right track and true reconciliation was possible. My optimistic feelings would not last long.

Once again, Nick left me without any warning. I was blindsided. When I thought everything was improving, my world would fall apart again. I felt all alone. I needed prayer and support, so I reached out to my group from the retreat to tell them Nick left me again. Chris was on the list of people I emailed asking for prayer.

REHAB, DIVORCE, AND MARRIAGE

2010 was a very busy year for me, to say the least. As you already read, I checked myself into a mental hospital and then a 90-day rehab after hitting an extreme all-time low and rock bottom. Nick divorced me while I was in rehab, begged me to return to him, and then left me again. Looking back, it was only by the grace of God that I survived all of this without trying to kill myself again.

With the help of social media, my life would quickly change. Yes, you heard me: Facebook brought a miracle into my life. I had deactivated my Facebook account when I went into treatment. I decided to reactivate after finally accepting that my relationship with Nick was over this time. I changed my status to single, and that is when I got a comment from some guy I barely remembered.

In all capital letters… "WHAT YOU ARE SINGLE???? I AM TOO!" was written on my newsfeed by Chris Owen. I had been through so much then that I didn't even remember who he was or how I knew him. I hardly recognized his profile picture because he had lost a bunch of weight and looked ripped, muscular, and super-hot. Not that he wasn't good-looking when we first met over a year ago, but he was next-level good-looking in his profile picture. I was absolutely attracted to him, and he was obviously interested in me from his comment.

I was a 29-year-old single mom of a three-year-old and an 8-year-old barely making it financially and emotionally. I had quit personal training, which was my gift but also a trigger for me that led me to destructive behavior. I was desperately trying to do the right thing and stay sober.

I found an office job that paid $9 an hour before taxes. Thank God, I had earth angels helping me financially because $9 an hour barely paid for anything. I was still a mess, but Chris was still pursuing me, so that was a win.

Chris and I started messaging back and forth with a lot of flirting. He lived 3 hours away from me. He tried to get me on the phone, but I used my kids as an excuse not to get on the phone with him. Messaging was way easier and more comfortable for me at this point. I was very guarded but also cautiously optimistic.

To my surprise, after a few days of messaging me, Chris was headed to see me. He lived three hours from where I lived. It made me feel special that he would drive all that way to see me. I had butterflies in my stomach when I opened my front door and saw him standing there in person. My fairytale dream felt like it was coming true. My prince charming had come to rescue me. I just knew it. I felt it all through my body. It was love at first sight. Well, actually, second sight, but you get the point.

Chris is a godly man, and he made it very clear from the beginning that he was doing it God's way this time because his way had not worked in past relationships. What did that mean? That meant he was not staying the night at my apartment, and we would not have sex. No sex before marriage was a new concept for me. No guy had ever had enough respect for me to even attempt no sex with me at first encounter, much less before marriage altogether. Let's be honest: I didn't have enough respect for myself to ever say no to sex.

He literally came in and swept me off my feet, and I did not make the no-sex before-marriage part easy on him. I equated sex with the love and attention I desperately longed for. Sex was not sacred to me by any means. I was twelve years old when this unhealthy behavior became engrained in me. I was almost 30 at this point. It would take a lot to undo what had been done to me at such a young age.

Chris stood strong despite me trying to tempt him many times. Looking back, I think I was unconsciously testing him. Did he really respect me? Could I trust him? Was he really the godly man he claimed to be? Could I manipulate him like I had most people my entire life to get what I thought I wanted and needed?

Praise the Lord, he passed my test and God's! There was a small caveat. Chris knew he probably couldn't hold out against my relentless pursuit for long. To my surprise, he proposed to me two weeks after that first visit in front of his whole family, down on one knee with a beautiful diamond ring in hand. Can you believe I had been married three times already and had never been formally proposed to? The whole experience was truly magical.

We got married about four weeks later in a small country church. We didn't tell anyone. We just did it. We didn't need anyone's permission or an audience. When you know, you know. We knew that God brought us together and that we were supposed to be together forever. We were married on December 17, 2010. Now, the real work would have to be done.

I wish I could say it was a happily ever after experience, but there would be many trials and another rock bottom before I would become the godly wife, mom, and woman God was calling me to be.

REFLECTION AFTER A YEAR OF SOBRIETY AND MY LAST ROCK-BOTTOM

Chris and I used to be all in with alcohol, unhealthy eating, and other destructive behaviors! We are "all-in kind" of people, especially me. I am all in if it's good, and I am all in if it's bad or self-sabotaging! I have had to learn to use my "all-in mentality" for good when caring for myself and serving others.

As I write this book, about a year ago, Chris picked me up from my stay at a thirty-day treatment center. Our fears and discomfort were running high even though we were excited and relieved to be back together. What was life going to be like without alcohol?

We had never been apart for that long and not under these circumstances. I let my guard down, and the devil had a field day. I told myself I wasn't really an addict. I could drink every now and then. I was still getting everything done and fulfilling my obligations and responsibilities. I thought! Have you ever rationalized or justified self-destructive behavior? I was the queen of rationalizing and justifying.

My PTSD and mental health issues had gotten the best of me. I was too tired to fight the battle in my mind any longer. So, my few drinks every now and then turned into binge drinking most nights of the week, leading to my fourth suicide attempt since I was sixteen.

I didn't really want to die. I just wanted the mental pain and torture in my head to stop. Please don't feel sorry for me. I am grateful for everything I have been through and done because it was all necessary to get me to this place where I can empathize with and help so many others struggling in silence.

My pain is my purpose. I would not change a thing. Chris and I have fought every single day this past year to be the people we are today that God has called us to be for His glory. I pray every night and ask God to use me as a vessel to further His kingdom. I ask him to bring people into my life that I can help.

If I can overcome addiction, trauma, and mental health struggles, you can too. Trust me. Shifting out of a victim mindset and getting your power back is possible. Living a life where you truly believe "life happens for me and not to me" is possible. Changing the narrative from "Why does bad stuff always happen to me" to "I am the dominant force in my life, and everything always works out for me is possible."

Yes, it will take a lot of dedication, discipline, drive, consistency, and work that feels uncomfortable and sometimes painful. Sadly, most people don't have what it takes. They quit when their motivation runs out, and it gets hard. I pray that I give you hope and inspire you by reading my story of what is possible when you do the work.

There won't be a lot of fast wins. Sometimes you will question if God really has a plan for all the crap you are enduring to get to the other side. It may take a year or two or more before you see the light at the end of the tunnel. Don't quit before a miracle happens!

Outlast the temporary pain and discomfort of growth, healing, and change. Embrace the obstacles and expect them to come. Embrace the suck one day at a time. You can do hard things! You have made it this far!

Behind every fear is the person you want to become. Fear is self-imposed. You alone create it, and you alone can destroy it. Fear can be destroyed, and it will come back as confidence. I don't know you or what you are going through or have been through, but I believe in you because I am not special. I am no different than you are. You, my friend, are one decision away from becoming the person God created you to be. What are you going to choose today?

CHAPTER ELEVEN

EXTREME GIVING & SERVING DID NOT FILL THE VOID!

WAS I A GENEROUS PERSON OR OVER-GIVER?

I have never really looked up the definition of extreme giver, but I have always referred to myself as one. Before writing this chapter, I thought I better look up what that meant. Wow! I was shocked to learn that extreme giving can be a rare form of narcissism. No one wants to be narcissistic, especially me. With that being said, I think there was a time I used my extreme giving as a form of manipulation to keep others attached to me because I was so desperate for love and attention, but I do not feel that way about myself now.

According to www.harleytherapy.co.uk, "It is really a question of our intent when it comes to giving. Real giving is done from a place of true generosity and because we have an excess of something to offer (time, support, energy). It tends to be an impulse we don't have to overthink. And the giving leaves us feeling good and energized." Being generous can be a very good thing. It is even biblical to give more than we receive. After researching, I can see why I was finding my self-worth in extreme giving, and it was largely due to my childhood trauma and fear of abandonment. If I gave and served as much as possible, they might love me enough not to leave me. "They" means all the people in my life and that I encountered.

Andrea M. Darcy, the author of Harley Therapy Mental Health Blog's article, "*Generous Person, or Over-Giver? Always Gift-Giving* says, "Over-giving tends to come not from generosity but hidden need. It is an energetic transaction where we expect a return, even if that is just praise, appreciation, or to stop feeling guilty. And when we give too much, we feel depleted, not energized. We might even feel annoyed at ourselves or with the other person. Over giving is often a sign of codependency. When we are codependent, we take our sense of self from pleasing others. So, we give too much to receive praise and attention, giving us a feeling of esteem. But ungrounded esteem does not come from within but from without."

Are you telling yourself and others that you are an extreme giver and server like me? If you are, you may want to look deeper into your motives and why you are giving and serving. I justified my behavior because I truly thought I was giving from a place of pure love, but that may not have been completely true. I found my self-worth from what I did for others and not from within.

I FOUND MY SELF-WORTH FROM EVERYWHERE BUT WITHIN

Do you find yourself searching for your self-worth everywhere but from within? Have you ever wondered why all your good deeds and accomplishments only made you feel good for a little while? I found myself relentlessly pursuing to give and serve on extreme levels as much as possible because of the amazing euphoric high I experienced after helping someone or achieving a goal. The problem was that the high only lasted a day before I crashed into depression again.

I had absolutely no idea how to find my worth from within or how to love myself. I have heard for many years to love myself and not base my self-worth on outside sources or what others think of me. That sounds great and all, but how in the heck do people do that? I just couldn't make that head-to-heart connection. I needed a road map because I only knew how to feel good about myself when I was helping someone or achieving which I have learned is a form of codependency.

Ever since I was a little girl, desperate for attention and love, I remember thinking I was never enough and nothing I did was ever good enough. The need to be perfect at everything consumed me, and when I didn't hit the target, I was aiming for, I would literally fall apart. I used to cry uncontrollably if I didn't get an A on a test, if anyone got upset with me, or if I didn't get my way. If I couldn't win or do it perfectly, I would not do it. I was not a fun person to play games with, to say the least. Does any of this sound familiar to you? I am pretty sure many of you out there are like me! I can't possibly be the only one with this issue.

After Chris and I got married, I knew I could not turn to alcohol and prescription drugs to change the way I felt. Even though I had several slips here and there with pills, I didn't stay in my addiction long because Chris would catch me, and I would get myself together quickly.

Looking back, I realize now that I was chasing that same high from drugs, alcohol, and relationships, but trying to find it in the healthiest way possible. Is there a healthy way to chase a high you can't sustain and doesn't come from within?

I found myself searching for ways to give and serve in extreme ways. God put it on my heart to give and serve, and I am always obedient when He puts something like that on my heart, but I was taking it to levels the average person would never even consider.

The bottom line is that I could not find my self-worth from my loving Father in Heaven. I did not understand what it meant to find my identity in Christ. I was chasing something I had no map for. I desperately wanted to feel God's agape love in my heart, but the feelings never seemed to come. I was lost, but God never stopped pursuing me. The time would come when it would all click, and I would make that head-to-heart connection, but not for a little while longer. I would have to experience a few more rock bottoms to finally get to where I always knew I could be, the woman God created me to be, to be used as a vessel to help further His kingdom in a mighty way.

WHAT DID MY EXTREME GIVING AND SERVING LOOK LIKE?

When I tell you I was an extreme giver and server, I am not kidding at all. It started with me giving above and beyond financially. I absolutely loved helping people in any way I could. Don't get me wrong, tithing is the biblical thing to do, and it was so awesome to be in a place where I trusted God with our finances. I was no longer holding onto money as I would never earn more. That was freeing.

When I became a full-time health coach and started contributing to our monthly income, I found so much joy in giving to random people and causes; I never tracked how much I was giving. What could be bad about giving so much you aren't tracking it? I am embarrassed to say my motive wasn't as pure as it should have been. I was filling a void in my heart that should have been filled in a different way. The satisfaction giving would bring me only lasted a little while, just like the high from drugs, alcohol, and food only lasts a little while.

Chris never really looked at how much money I was making or what I was doing with it. He trusted me. I wasn't buying things I didn't need or running up credit card bills, so he had no reason to look or be concerned.

One day, the Holy Spirit prompted Chris to examine my financial situation. We got into a huge argument when he called me out and brought it to my attention that I was giving away over forty percent of what I was earning in my health coaching business. I immediately got defensive. This was news to me that I was giving that much money away. What was the big deal? We weren't doing without, and all our bills were fully paid. Why in the world was he mad at me about this? I was extremely irritated.

I think God was using Chris to call me out at that moment, so I would look at myself and take a personal inventory. Was I giving out of obedience to God and because I felt like it was the right thing to do, or was I giving to make myself feel good? Talk about a gut punch!

Before I could give big financially, I went on as many mission trips worldwide as I possibly could. I had always wanted to serve in third-world countries. What was wrong with that? Well, the problem was I became addicted to going on these trips. As you have probably noticed, I don't do anything in moderation.

When I started going on mission trips, I was a stay-at-home mom of 2-year-old twins, a seven-year-old, and a twelve-year-old. My husband and family were super supportive of me going on these trips. Chris never once told me I couldn't go, no matter where the destination was. He believed if God put it on my heart to do something like a mission trip, who was he to stop me? That was a huge blessing.

I am so grateful that God allowed me and made it financially possible (I raised support for every trip I went on) for me to go worldwide to share the Gospel with the unreached. The problem was I was so distracted by the turmoil inside of me that I wasn't fully present at the moment when I was sharing the Gospel in these third-world countries. I missed out on a lot of what I believe God was trying to show me on these once-in-a-lifetime trips.

Sadly, I started using my mission trips to check out of my life and reality. I was using them like a vacation from my kids and mom duties at home. It felt so good to check out and not have to worry about anyone but myself for ten days. It was a win-win! I got a break from mom and wife duties, and I got to serve the Lord.

GOD USED ME TO SAVE A LIFE

How many people do you know that have given 65% of their liver to a stranger dying from cancer? If you said none, now you know someone that did. That's right! I donated the whole right lobe of my liver in 2018 to a stranger with liver cancer. I would do it again if the doctors would let me.

The big miracle wasn't me giving my liver away. What I want you to take away from this part of my story is the fact that God used someone as broken as me. He could use me even though I had abused my body with drugs and alcohol and tried to kill myself multiple times. I am still shocked by it, and I know without a doubt it was all God!

God had put it in my heart about eight years before my donation that I needed to be a living donor. When He first put it in my heart, I researched how to be a living donor like a crazy, obsessed person. Keep in mind I was full-blown into my prescription pill abuse.

When I was using addictive substances, I could not let it go if I got some idea into my head. Despite abusing prescription pills, I have always struggled with racing obsessive thoughts. I now accept I will be taking medicine for the rest of my life to keep this under control, and I am not ashamed at all about it.

I found a website for people like me who wanted to be living donors. The site matched potential donors with people needing an organ. They were extremely sick but not at the top of the transplant list. Most of them had lost all hope, and this was their last-ditch effort to get the transplant they needed to survive. Most of the people needed a kidney or bone marrow.

I just knew I would donate a kidney to someone one day! I was beyond ready and willing. That didn't stop me from drinking too much or taking pills. I guess I wasn't worried about the how. I just knew in my heart this was going to happen, so I registered on the website as a living donor.

I had a few conversations with people needing kidneys with the same blood type as me, but nothing ever panned out. After a couple of years, I put the crazy idea back in my mind and moved on to other crazy things. I stopped looking at the website to see if I matched with anyone and pretty much forgot about it.

God has His perfect timing! In 2017, out of nowhere, I got an email welcoming me to the matching donors website. I thought this was strange because I had been a member for years. This prompted me to check the site to see if I had any new matches or messages from people I was a match for.

To my surprise, I had a private message from a man from Kentucky needing a liver. What? I had never thought of donating a liver. Chris has told me about donating a kidney because I would probably need both kidneys. He never said I couldn't donate a liver. This is how my crazy mind thinks!

I quickly responded to the man's message, pretty much telling him I was all in. I was his girl. I would do whatever it took to give him my liver. He reminded me that this was not a movie. The process was much harder and more in-depth than me just saying yes. There would be a lot of testing that would have to be done before I could be considered. At this point, we only knew for sure I was a candidate because we had the same blood type.

There was also the issue of getting my sweet, supportive husband on board. Tony (the recipient) was a black man from Kentucky, originally from Nigeria. He was a Christian, so we would both pray about it. I bring up the fact that he is a black man because I think it's so cool how God brought me, a white stay-at-home mom, and Tony, a single man with no kids from Africa in his 50s. Such a God thing!

Fast forward, Chris was supportive. He believed that if God wanted me to do this, it would all work out; if He didn't, the door would be shut. I think Chris secretly thought there was no way this would end up happening.

I had to raise money for several trips to Chicago. That is where the surgery would take place. We certainly didn't have any extra money, and Tony was not legally allowed to help me out financially. The testing was intense, and there were many times I thought it wasn't going to happen. In case you are wondering, I had no problem not drinking alcohol when someone else's life depended on it. My liver had to be perfect.

Finally, the surgery took place on May 18, 2018. The surgeon said my liver was beautiful. This shocked me because of all I had put my body through. My addict mind immediately thought I must not have a drinking problem because my liver was beautiful. My drinking career would continue for a few more years.

God can use anyone, no matter what you have done or been through! Believe that! I am proof. All you must do is be willing and obey when He puts something on your heart. Don't worry about the how, God already has everything figured out for you.

Five years later, Tony is doing great and cancer-free. He is like family to me, and we have stayed in touch. He and his family mean the world to me. I am truly honored God picked me to be the vessel that saved Tony's life. I knew because of donating that God wanted to use me in a mighty way, but I still had some cleaning up to do before I could truly be used for His bigger purpose.

In the next four years, I would go through peaks and valleys like never before, which would prepare me for my mission now. God would whisper, "Keep going," when I could barely put one foot in front of the other some days.

CHAPTER TWELVE

From Rock Bottom to Breakthrough

I SIGNED UP FOR A DIET AND THINGS
WERE LOOKING UP

In September of 2019, my life dramatically changed because I said yes to what I thought was a diet. I was an almost 40-year-old momma who was tired, irritable, overweight (even though I was working out 5-6 days a week, 1.5 to 2 hours a day), depressed, hated what I saw in the mirror, uncomfortable in my own skin, not the wife or mom I wanted to be, and desperate to find a solution.

I started what I thought would be another diet I attempted and failed. To my surprise, I ended up feeling amazing almost immediately. I also lost 43 pounds in 3.5 months! My life was finally heading in the right direction, mentally and physically. This was my answered prayer and a miracle I never thought would happen.

After being a stay-at-home mom for about eight years, I decided to jump in and offer this amazing gift through coaching. I didn't realize how much I missed helping people get healthy. It had been a long time since I was a personal trainer, but my gift for helping people returned immediately. It felt unbelievable to be coaching others in health and getting paid for it. I was finally living the dream.

Chris even joined me on my mission to help as many people as God allowed through this life-saving health plan. We both got healthy, and everything seemed to be improving. I mean everything! We were in a growth mindset, soaking up all the mindset work we could do to be the best health coaches for our clients.

I was beginning to let go of my victim mindset, and my past hurts, hang-ups, and habits. I was so excited about life I let my guard down. We started traveling more and doing things we couldn't do before because of finances. Life was good until it wasn't.

MENTAL HEALTH ISSUES AND
ADDICTION SNUCK BACK IN

Chris and I were having so much "fun" in our new lifestyle that we began to partake in adult beverages way too many nights a week. I figured out quickly that if I was eating healthy, I could drink a lot of alcohol and not gain my weight back. Game on!

One was never enough for me. Chris could go to bed, but I would stay up drinking because I wasn't ready for the feeling to stop. I wanted to check on the stress I had created by being obsessed with growing my new coaching business. I was stressed and exhausted from chasing advancement in the company. Alcohol took the edge off. This started to cause problems in my marriage that I was blind to, and my mental health was going downhill fast.

Right before my final breakdown, I lay in bed most nights after having too much to drink, begging God to please let me go to sleep and not wake up. I was too tired to fight this battle that I had been fighting most of my life. I would wake up the next morning and do all the things I needed to do. I would go a couple of days without drinking just to prove I could then revert to binge drinking.

I had fooled myself into thinking I could stop taking my antidepressant because I had been doing all this mindset work since I started coaching. I had a good two weeks without it and quickly declined mentally.

Have you ever known what you needed to do to get out of the dark hole you were in, but you just weren't ready to do it? Have you been paralyzed where you just couldn't do the right thing? God told me exactly what I needed to do, but I ignored Him. I could stop when I was ready. I just wasn't ready yet. God always must get my attention in a big way.

I was drinking to help with my social anxiety when attending events. I had difficulty connecting with people if I didn't have some liquid courage. I was also stuffing unresolved feelings from my PTSD and justifying it all because I performed extremely well in my coaching business. These bad habits helped me cope. They served me at a time when I was not ready to let my walls down and heal. Alcohol served me until it didn't.

How did I return to this place of being out of control again? I never thought I would get to where I wanted to die again. Suicide ideations took a stronghold in my life, and pouring alcohol on it made it so much worse.

I was so desperate to stop this horrible cycle of self-sabotage. Something dramatic would have to happen to get my attention and bring my insanity to an end. I never imagined it would be another suicide attempt.

DARKNESS OVERTOOK ME

We become addicted to the familiar even when it doesn't serve us. Staying the same is comfortable and less scary than stepping into the unknown. I was in a dark place, unable to hear God's voice anymore because of my poor choices. Something drastic needed to happen for God to get my attention and draw me back to Him. I am so grateful He never stopped pursuing me.

On June 9, 2022, I hit my last rock bottom! Some hurtful events happened with some people very close to me leading up to this day. I guess you can say the wind blew the House of Cards over for me. I was so distraught from my hurt feelings that I binge drank for two days.

Chris had finally had enough. We fought, and he left the house for the entire night. In our 12 years of marriage, he had never left and not come back. One of my biggest fears was happening again. I couldn't take it anymore. The only way out for me in that moment was death. I stood in my kitchen and took a whole bottle of pills.

This was the final straw. Chris admitted me on a psychiatric hold, and I could not come home. He gave me the tough ultimatum of going to treatment, or I would lose my family. There was no question in my mind. I would do whatever he wanted me to do at this point. I needed help. I went straight to treatment one more time. This would be the beginning of my breakthrough and lasting change to be the dominant force in my life.

WHAT DOES LIFE LOOK LIKE SOBER

You may be wondering how I know this is my last rock bottom. Am I afraid of relapsing? My answer is if I drink again, I will die. Drinking alcohol and not taking my antidepressant medication is no longer an option for me. I look at it that extreme. I have to. Once I make my mind up about something, it's done. It is that simple.

As Chris was picking me up from my 30-day stay at treatment, our fears and discomfort were running high even though we were excited and relieved to be back together. What was life going to be like without alcohol?

We had never been apart for that long, especially not under these circumstances. I let my guard down, and the devil had a field day. My PTSD and mental health issues had gotten the best of me. I was too tired to fight the battle in my mind any longer, so my few drinks every now and then turned into binge drinking most nights of the week, which led to my fourth suicide attempt since I was 16.

I didn't really want to die. I just wanted the mental pain and torture in my head to stop. I'm grateful for everything I've been through and done because it was necessary to get me to this place where I can empathize with and help so many others struggling in silence. My pain is my purpose. I would not change a thing.

Chris and I have fought daily to be the people God created us to be and to use us as a vessel to further His kingdom. If I can overcome addiction, trauma, and mental health struggles, you can too! Trust me.

How did I stop this vicious cycle of being stuck in a victim mindset? Was it easy? No, but it had to be done. I had to be the wife, mom, and woman God created me to be, and that would not happen by staying a victim of my past traumas and circumstances. I was a Warrior, and from then on, I would do whatever it took to live that out. It has taken a lot of *dedication, discipline, determination, drive, consistency, and work* that feels uncomfortable and painful.

Sadly, most people don't have what it takes. They quit when their motivation runs out, and it gets hard. I pray to give you hope and inspire you of what is possible when you do the work. There won't be a lot of fast wins. Sometimes, you will wonder if things are ever going to change. Sometimes you will question if God really has a plan for all the crap you are enduring to get you to the other side.

Patience is a requirement. It may take a year or two or more before you see the light at the end of the tunnel. Don't quit before the miracle happens! Outlast the temporary pain and discomfort of growth and change. Embrace the obstacles! Embrace the suck one day at a time.

HOW DO I DEAL WITH THE DAYS THAT SUCK?

For every level, there is another devil... I still get stuck and paralyzed. It isn't as often, and I don't stay there as long now. I have new tools in my toolbelt to live life on life's terms. I no longer need the comfort of unhealthy substances to get through the hard days. I intentionally intercept old thoughts and behaviors that kept me feeling like a victim, and I flip the thoughts into a narrative that empowers me!

As I write this book, I'm approaching a year and a half of mental and physical sobriety! While that is a miracle from God, and I've put in a lot of work mentally and physically, I still have days that suck. Valleys and tough days are a part of life that I am grateful for today. They no longer paralyze me and affect my mood or day like they used to. I have to feel the feelings to move forward where I used to check out and numb the feelings.

Today, I am free of cravings (alcohol and pills are no longer an option), and I don't think about wanting to die. God saved me from four suicide attempts for a reason. I am on a mission to help as many people as God allows be radically transformed into who He created them to be through my story of *Wounded to Warrior* and my gift of empathy, connection, and compassion.

I have learned to put a time limit on my feelings of sadness, grief, self-pity, and other similar feelings. It is ok to feel this way every now and then. Some days, I have good reason, and some days, I have no idea why these negative feelings come over me. Giving yourself a time limit is key, in my experience. Talking to someone instead of keeping it inside is a great idea. When we bring darkness to light, it loses its power over us.

TO THE LITTLE GIRL WHO DIDN'T FEEL LOVED OR SEEN

I am so sorry you had to grow up so fast. My heart breaks for you. You deserved more. None of what happened to you was your fault. You don't know or understand it now, but God is preparing you for something huge. You have a purpose. Your pain has a purpose.

You won't have to perform or always be the best to get approval, attention, or love. You won't have to have sex with boys to feel loved. You are worth so much more, but every hurt and all the abuse you are going through will not be for nothing. I promise. You will see. Just keep going.

All of the tears and emotional outbursts will only be temporary. Keep going! Feeling like your heart is being ripped out of your chest every time someone says they love you and then they abuse you or leave you won't last forever. Hang on, your godly mate is coming. He will love you unconditionally and be in complete awe of you. Keep going.

I know you always felt alone, hated, used, depressed, crazy at times, hopeless, and so tired, but trust me when I say you were never alone. God was always with you, protecting you and loving you. You will see it one day. All of the times you should have died, He was there. He let you go through with the hopeless action but didn't let you die. He needed you. You will have so much good work to do once you get past this unfair trauma and begin the healing process.

Keep going; your pain is your purpose, and you will be able to help so many struggling just like you are now. It will all be worth it. God will not punish you for all the bad choices you are making along the way. There will be consequences, but these consequences are necessary for you to learn and grow. You will look back and say, that wasn't so bad. I needed that to become the person God intended me to be. You will be grateful for what the consequences taught you.

Just because you had an abortion, it doesn't mean you won't have children. In fact, you will have four beautiful children who love you and respect you no matter what. You will never have to feel alone again because God will bless you with a big immediate family, friends, and clients who will be like family to you. You did what you had to do at that moment. You really didn't have much say in it because your mom took you without giving you an option. God knows you were too tired to fight. He forgives you.

I know it feels like you can't do life without getting high or drunk to change how you feel because you feel so uncomfortable in your skin. You won't feel this way forever. You won't be more afraid of living than you are of dying forever. You can love life, live life, and cope without alcohol or pills. The cravings will go away. The stronghold addiction has over your life right now will go away. Trust me. Keep going.

Hang on a little while longer. There is an end in sight. An ending that is beautiful and glorious with healing and redemption. The end of your pain will be a new beginning and a life full of miracles. You will have such a connection with God that you will always feel the Holy Spirit. The feeling of God's agape love and the presence of the Holy Spirit will be better than any high you could ever get from alcohol or drugs. Trust me. Keep going. You can do hard things. Failure and setbacks are just another opportunity for growth.

This will be hard to believe right now while you are enduring the suffering and pain of all life has thrown at you, but you have been given a gift. The priceless, most valuable gift you have been given is empathy. Once you get to the other side of your trauma, God will use you as a sounding board to connect with others who are in the midst of a valley, feeling alone and hopeless.

You will feel the Holy Spirit as God uses you to see the struggling people. Not only will you see them, but He will use you to make them feel seen, heard, and comforted so they know they aren't alone. Your experiences are the qualifiers that will allow you to connect deeply with so many people from all over with different backgrounds. You will be used as a vessel to further God's kingdom just like you have prayed almost your whole life.

Don't grow weary. Like Damon West says, "*You don't have to win every fight, but you have to fight every fight.*" Remember to focus daily on getting 1% better than you were the day before. This will lead to monumental transformation over time. Trust the process and enjoy the miracles that are waiting for you on the other side. They are coming, so keep going.

CHAPTER THIRTEEN

HOW TO PARTICIPATE IN YOUR OWN RESCUE!

I am so excited to share some action steps with you that have been my game-changers. Everything I am about to share with you has helped me overcome my victim mindset to become the dominant force in my life and the woman God created me to be. I pray you take these steps seriously and implement them in your life. God will give us everything we need, but it is up to us to act and participate in our own rescue! We must do our part.

ACTION STEPS

1. Decide enough is enough. Get completely fed up with doing the same thing repeatedly and expecting different results. Your new life has to start with a realization that what you are doing is not helping you but hurting you. Then, your journey can begin.

2. Be honest with yourself and ask God to reveal to you the things or people in your life that are no longer serving you or getting you closer to where you want to be. Get ready. You probably won't like what He shows you. Some people will have to go, but God will replace them with healthy people who will be a blessing. For me, it was abusive people in my life, alcohol, and nonproductive habits like watching TV and scrolling social media. You will feel so much better when you do the hard things and eliminate what is holding you back. If I can do it, you can, too, trust me!

3. Have a baseline of non-negotiables in place. You do these things every day, no matter what, even on your worst day. This means you don't negotiate with yourself about these things. Some of my non-negotiables are my morning routine, working out, my bedtime, and eating healthy. I also turn my phone off an hour before I go to

bed and put it outside my bedroom when I sleep (a game changer). Stop negotiating with yourself. When you make a commitment to yourself, honor that commitment and build trust with yourself just like you would do with a friend or loved one.

4. Create a solid morning routine. Get up early. Successful people do not sleep in. I used to love sleeping in, but now I have disciplined myself to get up around 4:00 every morning. Why is this important? How you start your day sets the stage for the entire day. I have uninterrupted quiet time with God when I get up that early. I also write a declaration/affirmation paragraph and meditate on what I have written, and all the good God has done in my life. I quiet myself in peace and live in that place.

5. Be mindful of what you are eating and drinking. What you are fueling your body with affects every aspect of your life. Junk in, junk out, as well as health and mental issues. I contend for my health daily by eating a low glycemic, low sugar, high protein, low carbohydrate diet, which has completely changed my mind and body. I want to perform like an athlete, so I must eat like one.

6. On bad days, take action! Any action is better than no action. Not doing anything will only make you feel

worse, it will reinforce how awful you feel about yourself. It can be doing something as small as making your bed (which I highly recommend being one of your non-negotiables). Go back to your baseline! What were those non-negotiables that you promised yourself that you would do? When you struggle with being consistent, it is normally a lack of self-worth. That lack of self-worth comes from continually breaking the promises you make to yourself. One of the quickest ways to feel better about yourself and your day is to follow through with the commitments you have made to yourself that are leading you to the best version of yourself especially when you don't want to. I also want to encourage you to get outside of yourself by being of service to someone else. How long has it been since you randomly checked on a friend or loved one and told them they were in your heart? If you can't remember, it has been too long. Go ahead and do it now. Pick three to five people, send them a text or, better yet, a voice text telling them you are thinking about them. Ask them how they are. Ask them if you can do anything for them. Your reaching out may be the one thing that changes the trajectory of their bad day. How awesome would it feel to be that for someone else? Lastly, you don't need to be alone on a bad day. Tell someone you are struggling. Bring darkness to light by sharing what you are going through with someone you trust. When you share the darkness, it will lose its power over you. They may be going through something similar, and it will be good for both of you to not feel alone in your struggles. Not feeling alone is so powerful and comforting.

7. Self-care? What are you doing for self-care? Self-care looks different for everyone; it doesn't have to cost you anything. First and foremost, never feel guilty for taking care of yourself first. You cannot pour from an empty cup. You are no good to yourself or anyone else if you aren't taking care of yourself first. For me, self-care is simply taking a day off from working. I completely unplug, put my phone on do-not-disturb, and out of my sight. I remind myself as many times as I need to that there is nothing real but this present moment. Saying those words to myself helps ground me when my mind starts racing to everything I am not getting done or think I need to do. I also take a hot Epsom salt bath with essential oils like lavender and eucalyptus. I get a pedicure, manicure, or massage. I do a guided meditation almost every morning after I write my affirmation. I work out at the gym or run bleachers at

the local high school in my town (my daily form of self-care). I write my affirmation/declaration paragraph again. I enjoy hot herbal tea, coffee, or my favorite mocktail (two tablespoons of Apple Cider Vinegar, 1 scoop of pure ionic fizz magnesium plus, and topo chico or bubbly or LaCroix in a pretty glass). Another thing I love doing for self-care is going outside to enjoy God's presence as I look at and really take in the beauty of a sunrise and sunset. I find myself getting lost in the magnificence of His creation. If you are struggling with finding ideas for self-care, I recommend you google self-care ideas. You will get countless outside-the-box ideas.

8. Celebrating the victories is my favorite action step! This is an exercise I require all of the clients I coach to do on a daily basis. Every night, right before you go to bed, reflect on your day and all the wins you had. If you are saying to yourself, "My day was horrible. I didn't have any wins." You can change the narrative by asking yourself these questions. Take the bad parts of your day and ask yourself, "What did this make possible? What did I learn?" Now it is a win! I am a performance-driven person and sometimes get caught up in the unhealthy trap of always trying to be an overachiever. Celebrating small wins is extremely challenging for me. Not

acknowledging the small victories has not served me well so I am very intentional about celebrating myself for even the small wins now. Those wins may be that I got out of bed when I didn't feel like it. I made an appointment and went to it. I didn't lose my patience with my kids or husband. I bought groceries, paid bills, ate healthy all day, drank all my water, etc. A win is a win! Celebrate yourself daily whether it is big or small! You deserve to be celebrated. I have my clients write down three wins, they accomplished for the day and three wins they plan to get tomorrow right before bed every night. The idea is that we are going to bed grateful and happy with our accomplishments for the day on our minds. The purpose of writing down the wins that we plan to get tomorrow before we go to bed is to wake up with those wins on our mind and then we are more likely to make them happen. What we focus on grows. What we think about we bring about. Let's focus on the wins! I highly recommend you have an accountability partner for this step that you share your wins with every night. You are more likely to write your wins down if you know you are going to have to share them with someone else. Accountability is key to success in most areas of our lives.

Now, Let's Circle Back Around to That Daily Declaration/Affirmation Paragraph

I write mine daily and believe it with my whole heart. I didn't believe it when I first wrote it. I wanted, even dreamed, of a life filled with the attributes I list below. Every day I wrote it with trepidation, but I did it anyway. Today it is who I am and who I will become.

There is power in your words. And, when you declare who you are and what you want to be, everything in your life begins to align with your words and beliefs. Your behaviors change for the good. And your hopes and dreams are fulfilled day-by-day.

Here's mine:

I'm a positive, joyful, confident, empowered, highly favored, warrior, limitless, wealthy, impactful leader, spirit-filled, and godly woman with mountain-moving faith. My peace, self-worth, security, and value are in Christ. I'm a fruitful, sought-after public speaker, best-selling author, and coach with the ability to empower others to be radically transformed into the person God created them to be. I'm a magnetic leader who attracts highly self-motivated people who follow my lead. Abundance, favor, and wealth flow to me. Influential and prominent people who will help me achieve my goals come to me. I'm a relentless, perseverant, and lucrative best-selling author, public speaker, and life coach that everyone signs up with and aspires to be like. I expand in abundance, success, and love daily as I inspire those around me to do the same. I'm always in the right place at the right time. My husband looks at me with awe. My kids love and respect me. I look like a fitness model and train like an athlete. I pivot easily. I am the dominant force in my life. Everything always works out for me. I can do hard things!

Here are a couple of other examples:

I am clear on who I am. I am strong, bold, and brave. I am a leader. I am a chain breaker. I am "The One" in my family. I am valuable. I am worthy of all God has for me. My worth is not found from the people in my life or what I do. I am enough. I am learning and growing every day. I am a powerhouse. I love to exercise and push my body out of what feels comfortable. I am loved and appreciated by my husband. He showers me with affirmation, and we work together as a team. I am a mom who fights for her children.

My children feel seen and heard by me. I give myself permission for my voice to be heard, not being concerned with hurting someone's feelings as long as I am coming from a place of love. I am assertive and ask for what I want with no apologies. I am diligent and consistent in my relationship with God. I hold myself to a higher standard and rise to any challenge. I am excellent at helping others. People want to work with me. I love to start conversations and help people feel seen. I am creative and have vision.

— Kaycee Wiggins

I am a positive, patient, consistent, level-headed, financially stable, spirit-filled woman who makes others feel seen and valued. My life is filled with peace and balance. I create lasting friendships and real connections. People value my opinion and seek my advice personally and professionally. I excel in all my professions, am well respected as an expert in my field, and have gained wealth and financial stability for myself and my family. I am a strong, logical, intelligent woman people seek for mentorship. My husband and I are partners who share love, respect, intimacy, and workload. My kids love, trust, and respect me. My family and I are a team that works together towards our goals. I train like an athlete who loves and forgives my physical flaws. I pivot easily. Everything always works out for me. I do not sacrifice what I want most for what I want at the moment.

— Courtney Harrington

How to Write Your Declaration/Affirmation Paragraph

1. You must be very honest and vulnerable with this first step. You are laying the groundwork to create a new narrative about yourself. Get a piece of paper, a journal, or use the space provided below! Do what I call a "brain dump" and write all the negative things you say to yourself or think about yourself on a regular basis. We all do what I call "negative self-talk," which can sometimes play on a loop. You may ask a loved one you trust to help you with this part. Most of the time, we put ourselves down so often that we are not conscious of what we are doing, which crushes our self-worth and confidence.

2. Next, write down at least five adjectives that describe you at your worst. And the person that you don't want to be?

3. Now for the fun part! Take those negative statements and names you call yourself and flip them into positive affirmations. Ask yourself, "What if the opposite were

true?" about each statement. For example, the negative statement may be, "I am fat and ugly." To flip that to positive you would say, "I have a healthy and fit body, and I radiate beauty inside and out." Another example may be, "I will never be successful, and I never follow through with anything." To flip that, say this instead, "I am extremely successful at everything I set out to do, and I am consistent and dedicated, always following through to completion." Be bold! Dream Big! If failure was not an option, who is the best version of you and how would you describe her/him? I know this may seem silly, but please trust me. It works! I have been writing my paragraph every day for years, and now I truly see and believe I am all of those things I write in my affirmation paragraph.

4. Write down at least five adjectives that describe who you are when you are your best. These will go in your affirmation paragraph.

5. Include some dreams and goals that are so big you have no idea how they are going to happen, but they are your heart's desire. God put them there! They are possible. Write them in your paragraph like they already happened. You are declaring you are already your future self!

6. Add at least three to five mantras that motivate you and change your energy to positive and driven at any given moment. For example, mine are, "I am the dominant force in my life," "I pivot easily," "Everything always works out for me," and "I can do hard things." Feel free to use mine if you can't think of any yet. I say these to myself every day, especially when I am in a difficult situation.

7. Do not skip this step, ever! This step is one of the most important steps to changing how you think about yourself and your life. Consistency is an absolute must if you want this tool to help you step into the person God created you to be. I know you want that for yourself, or you would not be this far into my book! After, you have completed your paragraph, (remember, it doesn't have to be perfect! It will not be graded. This is for your eyes only. Set aside a time of day, preferably first thing in the morning, to write your paragraph. You don't have to feel like it, and you most likely won't feel like the new person. That takes a little time and lots of repetition. Feelings are indicators, not dictators! Just write the paragraph! Trust me! It works!

8. As time goes by and you establish this new life-changing habit of writing your paragraph every single

day no matter what, you may want to add to it or change it up a bit. It is a living document. It will evolve over time as you learn more about yourself, who the best version of you really is, and as God puts things on your heart to add to it. Trust that voice that says "You can dream a little bigger." Write down the scary goals and big dreams. Anything is possible, and you are worthy of everything God is putting on your heart."

Now it's your turn!

_____

_____

_____

_____

_____

_____

_____

_____

_____

_____

_____

_____

_____

_____

_____

_____

_____

_____

_____

_____

_____

_____

_____

_____

_____

_____

_____

_____

_____

_____

_____

_____

_____

_____

_____

I challenge you right now to make writing your paragraph every single day a priority, no matter how you feel or what you think about yourself today. Consistency is the key.

One thing I know for sure is that your opinion of yourself will change, your outlook on life will change, your family and friends will see the change, and you will realize every hope and dream that God put in your heart.

I promise!

TESTIMONIALS

Before reaching out to Tiffany for help, I had slipped backward into old habits. The fear that I felt envisioning myself losing all of my progress weighed heavy on my mind. Getting myself under control was something I didn't feel like I could do alone. Even in a thinner body, I was sad at the damage my choices had done to my health. I wanted to feel confident, and I knew that could only come with building strength mentally and physically. I couldn't imagine the type of support and encouragement I received through Tiffany's coaching approach. I look forward to working out now and realize that celebrating my body and strength makes a difference by setting aside time for me. No matter the setbacks I've experienced, Tiffany finds a way to encourage and reframe the narrative. I thank God daily for Optavia because it led me to the next step of my journey with Tiffany, who has coached me to success.

— Courtney Harrington

I want to let individuals know that YOU CAN achieve your goals, hopes, and dreams—no matter your age, circumstances, level of knowledge, or even despite your past experiences.

I partnered with Tiffany after I had released 106 pounds in a little over 9 months on an incredible health plan. I accomplished an amazing goal; however, I never exercised. I was over 50, and I kept the weight off, yet I became unhappy with the way my body looked — sagging skin, no muscle definition, and very little strength.

My previous fitness was littered with pain; personal trainers were either happy that I was nauseated and on the verge of throwing up or pushing me to the point of physical pain.

I desperately wanted to gain strength and muscle definition, yet I was terrified of reliving those experiences again. I shied away from asking for help, which only deepened my mental shame when I saw my reflection, which filtered into my relationship with my spouse as well as depleting my self-confidence. Yes, I had lost a significant amount of weight; however, deep down, I was drowning in shame, and that continued for two years until I reached out to Tiffany.

I had been watching her health and fitness journey for years. Although skeptical when she posted about taking fitness clients, I was intrigued. I wasn't an athlete nor athletic in any sense of the word; I didn't want to look 'bulky' or become a bodybuilder, nor did I want to endure pain or failure. I had already discounted myself before we even met for a consultation.

My whole world pivoted as soon as we met and has never been the same since. She met me where I was, listened to my past experiences, validated my feelings, designed workouts FOR ME, FOR MY abilities, NEVER asking for me to push myself past where I was physically or mentally able to go. Was I challenged? YES? However, she held me accountable to MY goals and my desires, EMPOWERED me to change the limits I had placed upon myself, and showed me how I can CONTROL my own story.

Six months ago, I thought I was partnering with a fitness instructor; I have found a life partner, a mentor, a friend, and a person who cared about me mentally and physically. Someone who helped me blossom into a confident, empowered, and resilient woman I didn't even know I could be. But she did!

My body has transformed. I have developed muscle tone and increased muscle strength. Now, I LOVE the reflection I see in the mirror daily.

I have learned so much through her mindset work and no longer allow the strongholds of my past to keep me from developing into the woman I am meant to be. At the time of this testimonial, I was 53 years old and in the BEST shape of my life. I have uncovered a passion for fitness, working out, healthy motion, and finding ways to challenge myself physically. I am a DIFFERENT woman than when I started. I am now in control of my destiny, authoring a story I never dreamed was possible that has filtered into every aspect of my life and relationships!

My story isn't over, and I have Tiffany to thank for unleashing and unlocking this new, vibrant, and healthy author that I have become in my life!

— Sara Tidwell

"When I die and meet God, I want to tell Him I did my best." I had watched Tiffany for a while. I saw her on Zoom and at a few Optavia events. As I watched, she became more and more of an aspiring person. Right from the beginning, I noticed that she possesses many qualities that few people have, qualities I wanted to build in myself. I first saw how disciplined she was in her workout regimen and her nutrition— never faltering month after month. But as I kept watching, the layers started to unfold even more greatness. Just a sparkle in her eyes when she looks at Chris on a Zoom chat or how she beams with pride talking about her children. It was easy to see and feel her love for her family. I also saw her as a human who made mistakes but could rise above it all and conquer life. I saw how much she leaned to God for help and deliverance. To become the best version of myself, I needed to plug into whatever this lady was doing!

I nervously messaged her and instantly felt a connection. I was worried at her level of greatness (in my mind) that I would hardly be worth her time, but here we are, six months later, and I can assure you, I have never once felt like I was the lesser person. Tiffany has the gift of helping you discover your true inner greatness! She makes fantastic workouts, but her ability to get you to your next best level both physically and mentally supersedes what I could have thought possible.

My life can be busy as a mom to an infant and toddler. With Tiffany's help, I have found time for me again! I have enjoyed working out when before it seemed a daunting task that never went away. I am waking up early (I am never a morning person) and have some structure back in what once was chaos. I am feeling even more positive and high on life (which is fun for me because I was already very positive, but this energy is next-level greatness!) I reach outward when I hit a stumbling block instead of keeping it all inside. Most of all, I've deepened my connection to God and can feel His love for me and all of God's children.

Thank you, Tiffany, for continuing to help me achieve my goal to become more like Him. Your strength, example, friendship, and pure love are inspiring. We are worthy. Life is beautiful. Let's keep going!

— Eliza LaCour

Where do I even begin? I decided to reach out to Tiffany in February 2023. I had lost 50 pounds with Optavia but had not yet reached my goal. I felt stuck, tired, and unmotivated. I knew I needed to work on my mindset, but I also knew I couldn't do it alone! I needed someone who had drastically transformed their life and mind to coach me on doing the same! I needed someone who would teach me to lean into discomfort and strive to be the dominant force in my life! Tiffany is that person!!

I was so nervous about our first Zoom consultation. I had not worked out in over three years and had significant anxiety about exercise. I also suffer from chronic back pain, which is one of the leading causes of my stress around working out. In the past, I have been made to feel like I would never be able to keep up or be fit. So, coming on Zoom to meet Tiffany had me feeling very apprehensive. Boy, was I wrong! She was all smiles. She was so excited to help me level up, build muscle safely, and address my mindset with anxiety. She made me feel seen. And she has helped me take charge of my fears and anxiety! Her workouts are challenging and effective. She designed my workouts around my ability, challenged me, and believed in me when I didn't believe in myself.

Because of her mindset coaching, I am where I am today! The workouts are unique, but the mindset coaching has transformed me!! I constantly get compliments from friends and family on my positivity and confidence and how much I've changed!

I've got back to teaching this year, and it's been the smoothest, least stressful start to a school year I've ever had. And it's not because teaching is less stressful it's because Tiffany has taught me how to manage my mindset! Life-changing!

And when I let life get in my way and the excuses accumulate, she continues to show up for me, and I feel supported and loved. I didn't know Tiffany before she began coaching me, and now she's a dear friend and mentor! She is the first person I think about when I have a win to share! She is the voice in my head telling me that I'm the dominant force in my life. She believes in me! I'll be her client until she retires! I'm now down 75lbs and counting!! I can't begin to express how much Tiffany has changed my life. And then, in turn, changed my family's lives! I'm forever grateful for her!

— Shawna Freeman

I watched Tiffany's FB posts and fitness client testimonials for several months, but when I saw her at the gym, I KNEW I had to reach out! I've always had a toxic relationship with exercise, cardio, and eating. I fed or starved my body and adjusted my workouts accordingly. I came to Tiffany for a fitness plan ONLY, and she saw straight through my BS. Tiffany knew from our first conversation that I needed a nutrition program, an intentional fitness plan, and a total mindset transformation.

I've always been willing to put in the work, BUT I was SO lost and needed accountability, a team, and someone to believe in me! I started on May 4th, and the rest is history. I did that first workout six days in a row and could barely walk. I've never been that sore in my life! A few podcasts in between while logging my food, and then came that 2nd workout and so on.

It quickly became a HABIT! Zoom check-in, log food, send my wins, listen to a podcast, weigh, new workout, participate in team challenges, A-team Zoom, see the scale move lower, fit in more petite jeans, long lost muscles started popping up, more energy, better sleep. Repeat! What?!?!?! I'm on #8 workout and have run over 30 miles this month because I CAN, not because I have to. I've worked out 80 TIMES since starting with you 112 days ago!

I don't even recognize that girl who messaged you in May in total desperation. She's different. She's gone. She's better because you believed in her, saw her potential, and made her believe in herself again.

— Casie Lewis

ABOUT THE AUTHOR

Tiffany Owen is a life, fitness, and health coach on a mission to see people radically transformed as she empowers them to be the best version of themselves. Her pain became her purpose. She's overcome PTSD, a lifelong battle with mental health issues, and addiction.

With 20 years of experience in the fitness and health industry, she is a voice for those suffering from a victim mindset that keeps them stuck in the vicious cycle of self-sabotage. She offers her experience, strength, hope, and inspiration to set them free! Her life's focus in life is to help others transform their minds, bodies, habits, and goals.

Let's work TOGETHER to create the lifestyle you envision and need to become the dominant force in your life.

READY TO TRANSFORM YOUR LIFE?

Get more Information

BOOK TIFFANY TO SPEAK

Hire for Speaking QR

www.ingramcontent.com/pod-product-compliance
Lightning Source LLC
Chambersburg PA
CBHW071152130626
46553CB00004B/1619